HIDDEN AGENDA:

PRESIDENT TRUMP'S FUTURE WAR ON CANNABIS

BY RUSSELL REDDEN

HIDDEN AGENDA:

PRESIDENT TRUMP'S FUTURE WAR ON CANNABIS

BY RUSSELL REDDEN

ISBN: 9798684308659

Independently published

HIDDEN AGENDA:

PRESIDENT TRUMP'S FUTURE WAR ON CANNABIS

By Russell Redden

Chapters

Preface..7

Introduction...9

Chapter One: **Actions Must Match Words**................................11

Chapter Two: **The Trump Administration Blocked Research**...............17
    A Lawsuit was Filed
    The New Cultivation Rule

Chapter Three: **The DEA Memo**...29
    Trump Tried to Keep it Secret
    The Text of the Memo

Chapter Four: **Reefer Madness at the Top**.............................43
    Trump Believes Cannabis Lowers IQ
    Rallying the Troops

Chapter Five: **Blocking Research Delayed Innovation**.................57
    40 Years and No Follow Up
    Asthma (Bronchodilation)
    Anticonvulsant
    Cancer
    Antibacterial Activity
    Sedative-Hypnotic Action
    Analgesia
    Antidepressant
    Cannabis Might Treat Covid-19
    Treats MRSA
    THC is a Possible Treatment for Alzheimer's
    How Many People Could be Harmed by Your Vote?

Chapter Six: **Trump's Donation Against Cannabis**.....................81
    The Surgeon General's Warning
    Higher Potency Strains
    Physical Dependence
    "Psychosis"
    Overdose
    Cannabinoid Hyperemesis Syndrome
    A Recent Phenomenon
    The "TRPV Channels"
    Deaths from Cannabinoid Hyperemesis Syndrome
    CBD Oil and the Mitochondria
    Cannabis and Heart Attacks
    A "National Threat"
    Pregnant Women
    Cannabis and Autism Rates
    Marijuana Use During Adolescence

Chapter Seven: **Behind The Scenes**...123
    Negative Input
    An Attempt to Block Cannabis Exports from Israel
    Will not Support Cannabis Businesses
    During Pandemic
    The Trump Administration Blackmailed Schools
    Over Medical Cannabis
    Immigrants are Immoral Who Use It
    Canadian Investors Banned for Life
    President Trump Opposes Access for Military Vets

Chapter Eight: **The "War" Between Cannabis and Opium**...................137
    Congress and the FDA Influenced by Pharmaceutical Companies
    Unethical Collaboration
    Conflicts of Interest in a "Cannabis-Heart Attack" Study
    The Beginning of the "Cannabis-Opium War"
    President Trump Doesn't Receive Any "Opiate Donations"?
    Opiate Influence, or Coincidence?
    Cabinet Positions

Chapter Nine: **Target CBD**..163
    President Trump's Anti-CBD Actions
    CBD is Technically Illegal
    FDA Warnings about CBD
    Statement by the World Health Organization
    The 2018 Farm Bill
    Regulatory Barrier
    HHS Petition
    Trump Requests Funds to Regulate CBD
    THC More Therapeutic Than CBD
    Pharmaceutical Money, World Health, and the European Union

Chapter Ten: **Vote Against the "Swamp" of Government Prohibition**...191
    Publicly Supported Corey Gardner
    Vice President Biden, Kamala Harris, and Cannabis
    Cannabis Prohibition Denies Transplants
    Harsh Prison Sentences
    Killed for Legally Possessing Guns and Cannabis
    Children Taken from their Parents
    The Effect on Drug Testing
    Physicians not Properly Trained
    Relocation Because of Federal Law
    Trump Cannabis Promise At Center of Feud
    List of Trump's Major Anti-Cannabis Actions
    Pandemic Relief Tied to Banking Reform
    A Vote for Trump is a Vote for a 2022 Republican Mid-term Disaster

PREFACE

Politicians make a lot of promises. At the same time, not every voter can keep up with all of the news. Many people have an important decision to make this November. If President Trump is reelected, the subject matter of this book will be tested. Based on the President's actions—combined with his personality—there is a good chance he is preparing to use current laws to shut down the cannabis industry. The ability to legally buy medical cannabis, recreational cannabis, and even CBD will be in great jeopardy in a second Trump Administration.

No one can tell the future, but all medical cannabis patients should be aware of Trump's anti-cannabis actions. No one should be tricked into voting against their own life, or livelihood. It it possible that even some avid cannabis advocates have missed news reports that reveal the true intentions of Donald Trump toward the industry. For reasons explored in this book, it appears the President cares more about a strict adherence to unjust, archaic laws than the lives of millions of people.

It is up to you after reading this book to decide if these conclusions are valid. Any politician will promise the moon to retain their power. Look beyond Trump's *promises* about this issue, spoon-fed in 30 second sound bites. Many of his supporters have heard these words, but are unaware of his actions on this issue. He has gone out of his way to block both cannabis reforms, and scientific research. Discover Donald Trump's "hidden agenda" against cannabis industry. His actions speak louder than his words.

Russell Redden
September, 2020

INTRODUCTION

For almost a century, Cannabis has been illegal in the United States. Due to prohibition, hundreds of thousands of people have not had legal access to this drug for some serious medical conditions. Many are in jail for small amounts of this plant, their lives ruined by the legal system. The black market is being well financed, earning billions of dollars from the marijuana trade. At the same time, the pharmaceutical industry has been giving millions of dollars to candidates to keep cannabis illegal.

Then suddenly, reforms began at the state level. The people of this country used their voting power to make cannabis legal, first for medical purposes, and later for adult consumption. Yet, despite the fact the American people overwhelming support these reforms, the President of the United States has been doing everything in his power against cannabis, blocking laws that would prevent the federal government from moving against the industry at a future time. This book lists scores of reports that together stack up as evidence of his true intentions.

For almost one hundred and fifty years, opiate money has corrupted governments, and these governments have spread "trumped up" claims against cannabis. THC is in direct competition with opium as a pain killer. The people corrupted with this money have continued to spread disinformation—the same tired charges, refuted by scientists every time they are made.

Current law allows the DEA to delay or block cannabis research, and government red tape by itself makes the scientific investigation of cannabis too costly. Because millions of people rely on this plant as a medicine, everyone should vote in the next election fully informed, to prevent a panned shutdown of the legal cannabis industry.

CHAPTER ONE:
ACTIONS MUST MATCH WORDS

*T*housands of Americans suffer from serious illnesses. At the same time, many of them are injured or killed from the side effects of legal prescription drugs. Preliminary research on lab animals indicate Cannabis could be a safer substitute for many drugs that treat these conditions. However, the majority of cannabis research in the United States has been difficult to perform since the Controlled Substance Act was passed. The CSA established a system of regulations that are used by government agencies to block the majority of *positive* cannabis research.

By standing in the way of recent reforms, President Trump proves he supports the status quo. These laws incarcerate people for exercising their freedom to treat their disease with a natural substance. Current law harms these people; without access to medical cannabis, some could die from some serious conditions. People who live in states unfriendly to cannabis have died, gone to prison, had their children taken away, and even been shot by police while sleeping. All of these things continue to happen, even in states with cannabis reforms. And, President Trump will likely "turn back the clock" even further, waging another "war on drugs."

Recent polls demonstrate why it would be in President Trump's best interest for his own reelection to support Cannabis reforms. As many as *two thirds* of the American people support the legalization of cannabis, and up to 90 percent support medical cannabis. From the *Pew Research Center*, we read:

> "Two-thirds of Americans say the use of marijuana should be legal, reflecting a steady increase over the past decade, according to a new Pew Research Center survey. The share of U.S. adults who oppose legalization has fallen from 52% in 2010 to 32%

today. Meanwhile, an overwhelming majority of U.S. adults (91%) say marijuana should be legal either for medical and recreational use (59%) or that it should be legal just for medical use (32%). Fewer than one-in-ten (8%) prefer to keep marijuana illegal in all circumstances, according to the survey, conducted Sept. 3 to 15 on Pew Research Center's American Trends Panel."[1]

If President Trump attempts to shut down the Cannabis industry after he is reelected, he will be in a small minority. Only 8% would support his actions. But if he believes he is doing right, he won't care. That is part of his personality. He surrounds himself with people who echo his fears about this issue, with selected information. They agree with his anti-cannabis beliefs, and are helping him do the exact opposite of his campaign promises.

When President Trump ran the first time, he stated clearly that he supported medical cannabis, and the right of each state to decide this issue. From *Brookings*, we read:

> "On the 2016 campaign trail, Mr. Trump didn't shy away from questions about marijuana. (It is worth noting that marijuana initiatives shared a ballot with Mr. Trump in nine states in 2016.) He noted in an interview with Fox News that he knew people who were helped by medical marijuana and that he supported it "100 percent," and suggested he was in favor of more research into the effects of marijuana. In another interview with a local Colorado television station, he noted that recreational marijuana policy "should be up to the states" and that he opposed federal intervention in legal states."[2]

These promises were spread throughout the media, and many trusted his words. He gave his voters the impression he wanted to reform these antiquated laws, allow access to medical cannabis, and let the voters of each state decide this issue. Yet each time he signs the budget into law, he wants to make sure he still retains the power to shut down the industry. This has been stated clearly by his Press Secretary. From Politifact, we read:

> "The Trump Administration signaled last week it could crack down on recreational marijuana in states such as California where voters legalized pot last November, marking a possible change from the Obama Administration's more permissive approach. "There is still a federal law we need to abide by in terms of when it comes to recreational marijuana and other drugs of that nature,"

<hr>

1 *Two-thirds of Americans Support Marijuana Legalization.* By Andrew Daniller. PEW RESEARCH CENTER. November 14, 2019

2 *Trump's 1st State of the Union: His chance to be a state's rights president* By John Hudak. BROOKINGS. Wednesday, January 24, 2018

White House press secretary Sean Spicer told reporters on Feb. 23, 2017. "I do believe that you'll see greater enforcement." The next day, Democratic California Lt. Gov. Gavin Newsom urged Trump in a letter to follow the hands-off pot approach he claimed Trump had promised during his campaign. "A Quinnipiac poll released yesterday says that 71-percent of US voters (say) that the government should not interfere with states that passed legalized marijuana and during your campaign, you committed to honoring states' rights when it comes to marijuana legalization," Newsom wrote on Feb. 24, 2017."[3]

The President's Press Secretary—without any rebuke from Donald Trump—*promised*:

"greater enforcement is coming."

As stated, President Trump wants to make sure he retains the power to shut down the cannabis industry. From *Motley Fool*, we read:

"Furthermore, President Donald Trump hasn't exactly thrown his hat into the legalization column. Although he commented during his 2016 campaign that he was "one hundred percent" in favor of legalizing medical marijuana, he's now appointed two attorney generals (Jeff Sessions and William Barr) who've strongly opposed to any sort of marijuana reforms at the federal level. Trump has even included presidential signing statements for legislation that pertained to cannabis. Presidents typically attach a signing statement to legislation that they feel may impede their ability to do their constitutionally mandated job. In effect, Trump's signing statement always leaves the door open for the federal government to impose its superseding law and clamp down on state-level cannabis industries."[4]

Three times when the President signed the budget, he made this statement. He wants to be on record that he still has the power to crack down on cannabis—but why? His words reveal his heart. Without any objection from the President, former Attorney General Jeff Sessions rescinded this rule:

"President Trump keeps flip-flopping on medical pot "For those who may not recall, Trump was in full support of medical cannabis

---

3 *TRUE OR FALSE: During his campaign for president, Donald Trump "committed to honoring states' rights when it comes to marijuana legalization."* By Gavin Newsom. POLITIFACT. February 24, 2017

4 *The Surprising Reason the U.S. May Be Reluctant to Legalize Marijuana.* MOTLEY FOOL. June 29, 2020

when questioned about the topic during 2016 presidential debates. He was quoted as saying that he was "100 percent" in favor of medical marijuana in the U.S. but opined that he'd need to see additional data before considering recreational weed for broad-based reform. However, this view from the president has undergone multiple transformations since 2016. For instance, not long after being elected president, Trump appointed Jeff Sessions to become his attorney general (Sessions resigned in November 2018). Trump was fully aware of Sessions' leanings, which included an ardent stance against the proliferation of cannabis in any form. In fact, Sessions attempted to persuade a few of his congressional colleagues to repeal the Rohrabacher-Farr Amendment in 2017. This rider (also known as Rohrabacher-Blumenauer) has been attached to all federal spending bills since 2014, and it's designed to disallow the Justice Department from utilizing federal money to prosecute medical pot businesses operating in legal states. Needless to say, Sessions' attempts to repeal this rider failed. Sessions was also responsible for rescinding the Cole memo on Jan. 4, 2018. The Cole memo, written by former Deputy Attorney General James Cole under the Obama administration, outlined a series of "rules" that legalized-weed states would need to follow in order to keep the federal government off their backs, so to speak. This included keeping marijuana away from children, as well as keeping cannabis grown in a legal state within that state's borders. At no point did President Trump intervene or speak out against Sessions' attempts to subvert the legal weed industry."[5]

After the Cole Memorandum was rescinded, President Trump "dropped a hint" that a crackdown was coming:

"Last week, President Trump might have dropped a hint about his thoughts on cannabis legalization. On August 30, Marijuana Moment reported that President Trump expressed his views. DC Examiner reporter Steven Nelson asked him about federally legalizing marijuana while he is in office. President Trump said, "We're going to see what's going on. It's a very big subject and right now we are allowing states to make that decision. A lot of states are making that decision, but we're allowing states to make that decision."[6]

President Trump said "**right now** we are allowing states to make

5 *Trump Continues to Flip-Flop on Medical Marijuana.* By Sean Williams, MOTLEY FOOL. YAHOO FINANCE. February 23, 2019
6 *Cannabis Legalization: Did President Trump Drop a Hint?* BY Sushree Mohanty MARKET REALIST August, 2019

that decision..." If you 'read between the lines,' Trump's is saying: "we are only tolerating this *now*." Compare these words, to the promise of his Press Secretary—"greater enforcement is coming." Similar words were spoken by Trump's campaign spokesman. From the *Fresh Toast*, we read:

> "Asked in a new interview about President Trump's position on changing federal marijuana laws, a top reelection campaign aide said the administration's policy is that cannabis and other currently illegal drugs should remain illegal."...Donald Trump previously supported states considering marijuana legalization, but that could be changing. Analysts previously predicted Donald Trump might support marijuana legalization to boost his chances of re-election this year. Instead, the opposite has happened. The Trump Administration has proposed removing medical marijuana protections in the 2021 fiscal budget and leaked audio revealed the President's belief that smoking weed makes you dumb. Trump has done little to reverse this appearance of an antimarijuana sentiment building in the White House. Rather, a top Trump campaign spokesman doubled down and said marijuana should remain illegal at the federal level...This complicates what Trump stated during his 2016 campaign and time in the White House. Previously, Trump supported leaving marijuana legalization to the states and voiced support for the STATES Act, bipartisan legislation that would prohibit federal prosecution for those living in states with legal cannabis."[7]

President Trump promised to support the STATES act, but has not kept his word. It is not possible to support these reforms, and believe Cannabis should be kept illegal at the Federal level. The STATES act supports giving people at the state level the right to craft their own cannabis policies. President Trump claimed to support this, but instead, it is likely he is only tolerating this "right now." When you read between the lines, this means there will be a crackdown later. After reading all of the reports in this book, you decided if this is a reasonable interpretation.

Why has no crackdown occurred yet? *The President is smart enough to know he should wait until after his reelection.*

---

7 *Trump Administration Doubles Down on Anti-Marijuana Position* By Brendan Bures. February 20, 2020 THE FRESH TOAST February 21, 2020

CHAPTER TWO:
THE TRUMP ADMINISTRATION BLOCKED RESEARCH

*P*eople all across this country are finding relief in medical cannabis—while the government denies any evidence of it's medicinal properties. This is because bureaucrats in our government have successfully blocked cannabis research. If a company wants to finance a study, but knows that it might take *years* to get approval—it is more economically feasible to study something else. These regulations, and laws all work in the favor of the pharmaceutical industry, which could lose *billions* if cannabis is legalized.

Even the Food and Drug Administration (FDA), and the National Institute of Drug Abuse (NIDA) recognize that regulations of the Controlled Substance Act have blocked research. Chuck Rosenberg, former head of the DEA, quotes their concerns. From the *Federal Register*, we read:

> "FDA and the National Institutes of Health's National Institute on Drug Abuse (NIDA) also believe that work continues to be needed to ensure support by the federal government for the efficient conduct of clinical research using marijuana. Concerns have been raised about whether the existing federal regulatory system is flexible enough to respond to increased interest in research into the potential therapeutic uses of marijuana and marijuana-derived drugs. HHS welcomes an opportunity to continue to explore these concerns with DEA. Karen B. DeSalvo, MD, MPH, MSc Acting Assistant Secretary for Health." [8])

The combination of regulations—and the power of the DEA—has

---

8 ***Denial of Petition To Initiate Proceedings To Reschedule Marijuana*** Federal Register Volume 81, Number 156. Friday, August 12, 2016

blocked, or delayed cannabis research for over 40 years. Many scientists have complained about this government interference, but the majority of the public is unaware it exists—or how important it is to remove it. Many trust their government to research these issues. Instead, it stands in the way. Two Governors have also petitioned the DEA reclassify cannabis, to no avail. From *Reuters*, we read:

> "The governors of Washington state and Rhode Island filed a petition with the U.S. Drug Enforcement Administration on Wednesday that would allow doctors to legally prescribe marijuana as a medical treatment. Democrat Christine Gregoire of Washington and independent Lincoln Chafee of Rhode Island are asking the DEA to reclassify marijuana as a schedule 2 drug from schedule 1 - where it is listed alongside heroin and ecstasy - which would make it legal for doctors to recommend its use and pharmacists to supply it."[9]

The DEA refused their petition. These denials continued to frustrate researchers. Until recent rules, they were only allowed to study marijuana grown at one farm in Mississippi. This cannabis was tested at only 2 to 8 percent THC—*only slightly more potent hemp*. This means that if scientists were finally given permission to study this plant, they received cannabis of extremely poor quality. From BioRXiv, we read:

> "Currently, the University of Mississippi, funded through the National Institutes of Health/National Institute on Drug Abuse (NIH/NIDA), is the sole Drug Enforcement Agency (DEA) licensed facility to cultivate Cannabis for research purposes. Hence, most federally funded research where participants consume Cannabis for medicinal purposes relies on NIDA-supplied product. Previous research found that cannabinoid levels in research grade marijuana supplied by NIDA did not align with commercially available Cannabis from Colorado, Washington and California. Given NIDA chemotypes were misaligned with commercial Cannabis, we sought to investigate where NIDA's research grade marijuana falls on the genetic spectrum of Cannabis groups... The purpose of this study was to examine the genetic relationship of Cannabis samples from the National Institute on Drug Abuse (NIDA) to hemp and drug-type samples. Our results clearly demonstrate that NIDA Cannabis samples are substantially different from most commercially available drug-type strains, sharing a genetic affinity with hemp samples in most analyses. Previous research has found that medical and recreational Cannabis from California, Colorado, and Washington differs significantly in cannabinoid

9 ***Two governors petition for medical marijuana*** REUTERS. November 30, 2011

levels from the research grade marijuana supplied by NIDA14 Our genetic investigation adds to this previous research, indicating that the genetic makeup of NIDA Cannabis is also distinctive from commercially available medical and recreational Cannabis."[10]

Many studies could be skewed because researchers used this low grade cannabis in smokable form. The samples provided by the government did not represent the majority of cannabis consumed, legal or illegal. Some of these samples were contaminated with yeast or mold. From *PBS*, we read:

"One sample, billed as having a 13 percent level of THC — the main psychoactive compound in marijuana — had just 8 percent when tested at the independent facility in Colorado. Other samples were off by lesser amounts. Subsequent testing at the University of Illinois-Chicago confirmed the presence of total yeast and mold. The Chicago tests also found all four samples contained trace amounts of lead, though well below the levels generally considered to be hazardous, at least for adults."[11]

Researchers complained about this low grade cannabis, and in response to their concerns, the DEA announced it would change it's policies. This new policy was posted a few months prior to the election of President Trump. On the *DEA* website, we read:

"To facilitate research involving marijuana and its chemical constituents, DEA is adopting a new policy that is designed to increase the number of entities registered under the Controlled Substances Act (CSA) to grow (manufacture) marijuana to supply legitimate researchers in the United States. This policy statement explains how DEA will evaluate applications for such registration consistent with the CSA and the obligations of the United States under the applicable international drug control treaty. ...There are a variety of factors that influence whether and to what extent such research takes place. Some of the key factors—such as funding—are beyond DEA's control.[2] However, one of the ways DEA can help to facilitate research involving marijuana is to take steps, within the framework of the CSA and U.S. treaty obligations, to increase the lawful supply of marijuana available to researchers. For nearly 50 years, the United States has relied on a single grower to produce marijuana used in research. This grower

---

10 *Research grade marijuana supplied by the National Institute on Drug Abuse is genetically divergent from commercially available Cannabis* BIORXIV. Anna L. Schwabe, Connor J. Hansen, Richard M. Hyslop, Mitchell E. McGlaughlin. August 3, 2019
11 *Scientists say the government's only pot farm has moldy samples—and no federal testing standards* By Caleb Hellerman PBS Mar 8, 2017

operates under a contract with the National Institute on Drug Abuse (NIDA). This longstanding arrangement has historically been considered by the U.S. Government to be the best way to satisfy our nation's obligations under the applicable international drug control treaty, as discussed in more detail below. For most of the nearly 50 years that this single marijuana grower arrangement has been in existence, the demand for research-grade marijuana in the United States was relatively limited—and the single grower was able to meet such limited demand. However, in recent years, there has been greater public interest in expanding marijuana-related research, particularly with regard to certain chemical constituents in the plant known as cannabinoids."[12]

After the DEA posted this policy change, nothing occurred for over three years. No new applications were approved. The Trump Administration had come into power, and the DEA now answered to Jeff Sessions. During President Trump's entire first term, the DEA "sat on" over 30 applications from companies to grow research-grade cannabis. From *the Hill*, we read:

"It's been nearly three years since the Drug Enforcement Administration formally announced plans to facilitate FDA-approved marijuana-related research in the United States. Unfortunately, in the 36 months since then, the agency has woefully to follow through on their pledge. In August 2016, the agency that it had a adopted a new policy "to increase the number of entities registered under the Controlled Substances Act (CSA) to grow marijuana to supply legitimate researchers in the United States." This policy change is necessary and long overdue. That is because under federal regulations dating back to the late 1960s, only a single licensed entity – the — is permitted to cultivate cannabis for clinical research purposes. This monopoly has stifled clinical investigations into the marijuana plant. Notably, the cannabis grown by the university is often of and typically fails to reflect the wide variety of strains and products commonly used by the general public. Specifically, a research analysis published earlier this year by investigators at the University of Northern Colorado that the program's marijuana strains more closely resemble industrial hemp (a low-THC variety of the plant grown for fiber content) than the varieties of cannabis commonly available in dispensaries throughout the country."[13]

12 *Applications To Become Registered Under the Controlled Substances Act To Manufacture Marijuana To Supply Researchers in the United States A Rule by the Drug Enforcement Administration* 08/12/2016

13 *Three years ago the DEA said they would remove roadblocks to cannabis research—they still haven't* THE HILL By Paul Armentano. 07/31/19

During Jeff Sessions tenure as Attorney General, everyone blamed him for this obstruction. Congress even questioned him about these delays. From *Brookings*, we read:

> "Last week, during a Senate Judiciary Committee hearing Orrin Hatch (R-Utah) asked Attorney General Jeff Sessions a question about cannabis. It wasn't about legalization or enforcement. It was about science. Sen. Hatch asked the Attorney General for a status update on applications to grow cannabis for federally-approved medical and scientific research. The Attorney General offered a weak response that highlighted his own biases on the issue, a division of opinion between him and the president he serves, and a federal government effort to stand in the way of the free conduct of research."[14]

This news report claims the Attorney General, and the President have a "division of opinion" about this issue. Looking back, this analysis does not appear to be correct. Sessions was not acting alone, but with the blessing of Donald Trump. Subsequent facts presented in this book will prove this is the case. This obstruction has continued with William Barr as Attorney General. Both men acted according to the instructions of their boss.

The new DEA rules were not implemented because President Trump took office. His legal team changed the DEA's course of action. Earlier this year, Congress asked the Administration to change these rules. From *the Hill*, we read:

> "House lawmakers are growing increasingly frustrated with restrictions on federal marijuana research and are putting pressure on regulators to change the rules. While 33 states have legalized marijuana for medicinal purposes, federal research is extremely restricted. During a House Energy and Commerce Health Subcommittee hearing Wednesday, bipartisan lawmakers pressed officials from the Food and Drug Administration, Drug Enforcement Administration (DEA) and National Institute on Drug Abuse about obstacles to studying the safety and effectiveness of cannabis products, including hemp-based cannabidiol. "States' laws and federal policy are a thousand miles apart. As more states allow cannabis, the federal government still strictly controls and prohibits it, even restricting legitimate medical research," said subcommittee Chairwoman Anna Eshoo (D-Calif.)."[15]

The Administration has now released the new rules for cannabis research.

---

14 *AG Sessions blocks progress on medical cannabis research*
BROOKINGS. Wednesday, October 25, 2017
15 *Lawmakers press Trump officials to change federal marijuana rules*
By Nathaniel Weixel THE HILL 01/15/20

If enforced, these new rules would keep CBD, and THC illegal, unless in a patented medication. Right now, no major actions are being taken against cannabis—likely due to political deviousness.

A Lawsuit Was Filed

After one researcher who received this poor quality cannabis filed a lawsuit to force the DEA to keep it's previous promise to allow more companies to grow cannabis for research. From *Law360*, we read:

> "An Arizona marijuana researcher has accused the federal Drug Enforcement Administration of dragging its feet for more than three years on granting licenses to grow cannabis for clinical studies, blocking more than 30 would-be cultivators and stifling medical research. The Scottsdale Research Institute is seeking a court order from the D. C. Circuit compelling the DEA to clear cannabis growing operations at medical research facilities, which for decades have been limited to using low-quality marijuana produced at the only federally sanctioned cannabis farm in the country."[16]

The court ruling ordered the DEA to explain this three year delay. From the report, *Marijuana Moment*, we read:

> "Due to this delay, a lawsuit was filed against the federal government. A federal court demanded the DEA explain the delay in these applications :A federal court is ordering the Drug Enforcement Administration (DEA) to respond to a lawsuit concerning the status of applications for research-grade marijuana manufacturers. Researchers filed a suit against the agency last month, arguing that the quality of cannabis supplied from the nation's only federally authorized cultivation facility is inadequate and that additional manufacturers are necessary to increase the diversity of marijuana for research purposes. DEA said in 2016 that it was accepting applications for such facilities but has so far declined to act on the dozens it has received. The Scottsdale Research Institute (SRI), which submitted an application to grow its own cannabis in order to conduct clinical trials on marijuana's potential to treat symptoms of post-traumatic stress disorder, is seeking a resolution through the courts. On Monday, the U.S. Court of Appeals for the D.C. Circuit handed SRI an initial procedural victory, issuing an order that DEA "file a response to the amended mandamus petition, not to exceed 7,800 words,

---

16 *DEA Blocking Medical Cannabis Research Licenses, Lab Says* LAW360 September 13, 2019

within 30 days of the date of this order." [17]

In response to this court decision, the DEA announced that a new rule was being crafted that would make the old rule obsolete. This subverted the court's ruling. From *the Hill*, we read:

> "The DEA in 2016 first announced it would consider granting additional licenses for marijuana growers in order to increase the supply of research-grade cannabis. The agency has since received 33 submissions but has not evaluated any of them. That delay prompted a lawsuit from the Arizona-based Scottsdale Research Institute (SRI), which was trying to study the effects of marijuana on treating symptoms of post-traumatic stress disorder. The company asked a federal court to force the DEA to explain why it wasn't approving new applications. In a subsequent court filing, the DEA said its intent to publish a new rule makes the lawsuit invalid." [18]

We will learn the delay was due to a legal decision by the Trump Administration. The DEA had announced this new rule *before* Trump took office, but never acted on it, because his Administration interfered. In March 2020, the DEA announced the new rule. From *C&EN Chemistry News*, we read:

> "In March, the US Drug Enforcement Administration released a new rule intended to allow more organizations to grow more varieties of cannabis, but the cannabis research community says the proposal is still too restrictive. Additionally, cannabis researchers face the need to get approval from three federal agencies, and funding is limited. All these obstacles hinder cannabis research, the community says, leaving medical providers and consumers in the dark about the benefits and risks of cannabis products. Researchers have complained for years about the quality and potency of the cannabis grown by the University of Mississippi. In general, it has lower levels of THC than products that are available in legal state markets, says Morgan Fox, media relations director of the National Cannabis Industry Association (NCIA), a trade group for the cannabis industry. Researchers have reported that the cannabis is moldy. Additionally, the material is "basically like powder," Fox says. "So it is not really representative of what people are actually consuming," he says. The cannabis grown by the University of Mississippi has the appearance of being poor

17 *Federal Court Orders DEA To Explain Marijuana Research Block*. By Kyle Jaeger. MARIJUANA MOMENT. July 30, 2019

18 *Trump DEA to move forward on new marijuana grower applications*. BY Nathaniel Weixel. THE HILL. 08/26/19

quality because it is highly processed. It is dried immediately after harvesting and stored for long periods of time, sometimes years, in a walk-in freezer at −20 °C."[19]

This "new rule" was based on instructions from the Trump Administration, in a memo circulated in the agency. This "new rule" only allows companies to investigate cannabinoids extracted from Hemp (under the guise of "cannabis research.") Trump's response to congresses request *has* opened the door to new research—*except for THC.*

The New Cultivation Rule

In crafting this new cultivation rule, this Administration appears to care more about United Nations protocols, instead of logical sense. *Cannabis must be controlled as the opium poppy.* From the *Federal Register*, we read:

> "The Drug Enforcement Administration is proposing to amend its regulations to comply with the requirements of the Controlled Substances Act, including consistency with treaty obligations, in order to facilitate the cultivation of marihuana for research purposes and other licit purposes. Specifically, this proposed rule would amend the provisions of the regulations governing applications by persons seeking to become registered with DEA to grow marihuana as bulk manufacturers and add provisions related to the purchase and sale of this marihuana by DEA.
> Under the Controlled Substances Act (CSA), all persons who seek to manufacture a controlled substance must apply for and obtain a DEA registration...Because marihuana is a schedule I controlled substance, applications by persons seeking to become registered to manufacture marihuana are governed by 21 U.S.C. 823(a). ...Under section 823(a), for DEA to grant a registration, the DEA Administrator must determine that two conditions are satisfied: (1) The registration is consistent with the public interest (based on the enumerated criteria in section 823(a)), and (2) the registration is consistent with U.S. obligations under the Single Convention on Narcotic Drugs, 1961...In 2016, DEA issued a policy statement aimed at expanding the number of manufacturers who could produce marihuana for research purposes. ...Subsequently, the Department of Justice (DOJ) undertook a review of the CSA, including the provisions requiring consistency with obligations under international treaties such as the Single Convention, and determined that certain changes to its 2016 policy were needed. The pertinent Treaty provisions are found in articles 23 and 28 of the Single Convention, which are

19 *Cannabis research stalled by federal inaction.* by Britt E. Erickson. C&EN. June 29, 2020

summarized below. Additionally, DEA believes that these changes will enhance and improve research with marihuana and facilitate research that could result in the development of marihuana-based medicines approved by the Food and Drug Administration (FDA)....Because the terminology used in the Single Convention is somewhat different from that in the CSA, a brief explanation is warranted. The Single Convention uses the terms "cannabis," "cannabis plant," and "cannabis resin"—all of which are generally encompassed by the CSA definition of "marihuana" in 21 U.S.C. 802(16)).(4)The Single Convention defines "cannabis plant" as "any plant of the genus Cannabis."... from which the resin has not been extracted."...Article 28 of the Single Convention states in paragraph 1: "If a Party permits the cultivation of the cannabis plant for the production of cannabis or cannabis resin, it shall apply thereto the system of controls as provided in article 23 respecting the control of the opium poppy." Paragraph 2 of that article excludes from the Convention the cultivation of cannabis for industrial or horticultural purposes. Because the United States permits the cultivation of marihuana for the production of cannabis and cannabis resin currently only for research purposes, it is obligated under the Treaty to apply to the marihuana plant cultivated for these purposes the "system of controls" provided in article 23 respecting the control of the opium poppy...The system of control over all stages of the drug economy which the Single Convention provides has two basic features: Limitation of narcotic supplies of each country . . . to the quantities that it needs for medical and scientific purposes, and authorization of each form of participation in the drug economy, that is, licensing of producers, manufacturers and traders . . . .In the case of the production of opium, coca leaves, cannabis and cannabis resin, this régime is supplemented by the requirement of maintaining government monopolies for the wholesale and international trade in these drugs in countries which produce them. . . ."[20]

So, the controls on cannabis *supported* by the Trump Administration treat cannabis "as the opium poppy," and *limits* cannabis cultivation for "medical and scientific purposes." It is impossible for the Trump Administration to take these new regulations seriously, and allow state cannabis programs to continue. Why did the DEA change this rule? *We are told*:

"Subsequently, the Department of Justice (DOJ) undertook a review of the CSA, including the provisions requiring consistency

---

[20] *Controls To Enhance the Cultivation of Marihuana for Research in the United States.* Federal Register. 3/23/2020

with obligations under international treaties such as the Single Convention, and determined that certain changes to its 2016 policy were needed."

What happened between 2016, and 2018? *The Trump Administration*. It was behind this rule change, which appears to allow more cannabis cultivation, but in reality keeps the same (or stricter) controls on THC, and only expands research into other cannabinoids. "Cannabis resin" is still controlled under U.N. treaties. We read:

> "Article 28 of the Single Convention states in paragraph 1: "If a Party permits the cultivation of the cannabis plant for the production of cannabis or cannabis resin, it shall apply thereto the system of controls as provided in article 23 respecting the control of the opium poppy." Paragraph 2 of that article excludes from the Convention the cultivation of cannabis for industrial or horticultural purposes. Because the United States permits the cultivation of marihuana for the production of cannabis and cannabis resin currently only for research purposes, it is obligated under the Treaty to apply to the marihuana plant cultivated for these purposes the "system of controls" provided in article 23 respecting the control of the opium poppy."

So, if CBD is considered "cannabis resin," it is illegal. And, if "cannabis" is grown for *any other reason* than industrial, or horticultural purposes (Hemp,) cannabis must be controlled as the opium poppy. These controls slow research, causing many companies to shy away researching cannabis. The DEA will still have control over these licenses, only with a catch. We read:

> "Thus, any person who seeks to plant, cultivate, grow, or harvest marihuana to supply researchers or for other uses permissible under the CSA (such as product development) must obtain a DEA manufacturing registration. Because marihuana is a schedule I controlled substance, applications by persons seeking to become registered to manufacture marihuana are governed by 21 U.S.C. 823(a). See generally 76 FR 51403 (2011); 74 FR 2101 (2009), pet. for rev. denied, Craker v. DEA, 714 F.3d 17 (1st Cir. 2013). Under section 823(a), for DEA to grant a registration, the DEA Administrator must determine that two conditions are satisfied: (1) The registration is consistent with the public interest (based on the enumerated criteria in section 823(a)), and (2) the registration is consistent with U.S. obligations under the Single Convention on Narcotic Drugs, 1961 ("Single Convention" or "Treaty"), 18 U.S.T. 1407.""

The Trump Administration has kept a barrier in place that is responsible for many of the delays in cannabis research. The DEA will still grant licenses—giving *them* the power to delay. Their decision must be based on two criteria: *the public interest*, and *obligations under the Single Convention on Narcotic Drugs*, a United Nations treaty. The DEA could interpret "the public interest" according to their own whim.

Some do not believe these changes will have any effect on legal dispensaries. There is a reason this logic is flawed. In the next chapter, we will discover these new rules are based on a legal decision the President tried to keep secret. This legal interpretation concludes the government must have a *monopoly* on all cannabis grown in the United States.

CHAPTER THREE:
THE DEA MEMO

As we learned in the last chapter, the DEA has delayed applications to produce research grade cannabis for the entire time of the Trump Administration. We now know that a memo written by Trump's legal team was behind this obstruction, not Jeff Sessions. As this was taking place, health experts at the United Nations were debating cannabis rescheduling. From *Forbes*, we read:

> "Global health experts at the United Nations are recommending that marijuana and its key components be formally rescheduled under international drug treaties. The World Health Organization (WHO) is calling for whole-plant marijuana, as well as cannabis resin, to be removed from Schedule IV—the most restrictive category of a 1961 drug convention signed by countries from around the world. ...WHO is also moving to make clear that cannabidiol and CBD-focused preparations containing no more than 0.2 percent THC are "not under international control" at all. It had previously been the case that CBD wasn't scheduled under the international conventions, but the new recommendation is to make that even more clear."[21]

If rescheduling would have occurred, the main argument of this Administration against cannabis reforms would have been undercut. We will discover this Administration has based all new cannabis rules on a *strict* interpretation of international treaties. Members of his Administration have voiced opposition to cannabis rescheduling in the UN Single Convention on

21 *World Health Organization Recommends Reclassifying Marijuana Under International Treaties.* By Tom Angell. FORBES. Feburary 1, 2019

Narcotic Drugs. From *Cannabis Law Report,* we read:

> "A vote on WHO's reclassification recommendations was initially expected to be taken up last year by the UN's Commission on Narcotic Drugs, where the body's 53 member nations would decide whether to move forward with them...While the document acknowledges that deleting cannabis from the Schedule IV of the 1961 Convention could be a "benefit to the advancement of collective knowledge of both the therapeutic utility as well as any associated harms" by promoting research, it expresses concern about unintended consequences such as giving people the impression that legalization will follow...The document goes on to say that the WHO's proposed scheduling change might give people the impression that the Schedule IV classification poses "inherent barriers to research" and that the international framework is "incompatible with such scientific research." In other words, despite recognizing the potential benefits that WHO laid out in its rescheduling recommendation, the U.S. seems to remain concerned about the optics." [22]

Despite admitting "barriers to research," this Administration is reported to worry more "about the optics." Is this true? Would they stand in the way of researching new drugs for the sick, because it might help the legalization movement? It is because they have a scheme to keep it illegal, based UN treaties.

The World Health Organization has put off a vote on rescheduling several times, and the Trump Administration joined with several countries to delay it *again.* From *CND Blog,* we read:

> "USA: We echo the statement of the EU and Canada. We join consensus on the decision to vote on the cannabis recommendations in December in order to allow member states and the Commission to share their views on the impacts. We recognize that there will be a diversity of viewpoints – this is important. We urge the CND and other states to study these issues throughout the intersessional period so all states are ready to vote in December. Not seeking to undermine the scientific evidence. The importance of the WHO critical review of cannabis should be put into perspective: this reaffirms the placement of cannabis in Schedule 1. This is a major milestone in our efforts to control narcotic drugs liable to abuse but having some potential therapeutic value. We cannot lose sight that the world drug problem is vast and multi-faceted. Much remains to be done. This

---

22 ***The Feds Are Worried International Marijuana Rescheduling Could Boost Legalization Efforts*** February 4, 2020. Alternate link.

cannot be sidelined by other deliberations, so the USA reaffirms its support to use these next 6 months productively so we are ready to vote in December."[23]

Some member states agreed to put off this vote to achieve a consensus. The US voted to delay it as well, but likely so it will be defeated. Now *suddenly*, the European Union has publicly stated they will vote against rescheduling CBD, giving the same excuse. From *Hemp Industry Daily*, we read:

> "The executive branch of the European Union is changing its stance on how EU countries should vote on the World Health Organization's cannabis scheduling changes in December, Hemp Industry Daily has learned. The development comes on the heels of the European Commission announcing its preliminary view that CBD extracted from the flowering tops of the Cannabis sativa L. plant should be considered a narcotic under a 1961 United Nations treaty. If the Commission's new stance is formally adopted, hemp-derived CBD would no longer be considered food, would fall outside the scope of the bloc's novel food regulation and could be banned from the EU market....While the commission's "treat CBD as narcotic" stance is itself not shocking, "it is extremely puzzling why they have come forward with this position now," said Eveline Van Keymeulen, a Paris-based attorney at Allen & Overy." [24]

Is it coincidence that they have changed their mind, using the same argument of the DEA memo? This vote on CBD is scheduled for December, as the vote to reschedule Cannabis. The fact that the European Union has announced they will vote *against* rescheduling CBD, reveals how they will vote on cannabis.

Trump Tried to Keep it Secret

After someone at the DEA leaked the existence of this memo, many requested its release. President Trump attempted to keep it secret, claiming executive privilege. However, the Scottsdale Research Institute filed a lawsuit, and it was released. From *MG Magazine*, we read:

> WASHINGTON, D.C.– The Drug Enforcement Administration (DEA) has been required to release an internal memo that was supposedly used to force delays in approving new cannabis manufacturers to conduct research into the plant. Under the Freedom of Information Act, the Scottsdale Research Group,

---

23 *Item 5. Implementation of the international drug control treaties (continued)* CND BLOG. March 4, 2020

24 *EU Commission revises stance on WHO cannabis scheduling vote as it leans toward CBD as a narcotic* By Monica Raymunt HEMP INDUSTRY DAILY. July 30, 2020

an organization seeking to cultivate cannabis for research, filed a lawsuit last month accusing the DEA of using a secret memo as justification for not approving additional manufacturers to cultivate cannabis. This week, a settlement in the case h reached. The DEA released the memo in question as part of the settlement agreement. Although a settlement was reached, the DEA claims it is not admitting they violated any law. "The parties acknowledge that this Settlement Agreement is entered into solely for the purpose of settling and compromising the claims in this action without further litigation, and it shall not be construed as evidence or as an admission regarding any issues of law or fact," the DEA said in the agreement."[25]

The government settled out of court, and the document was released. Why would President Trump attempt to classify this document? It proves his campaign promises about cannabis are a fraud. But beyond this, it's details reveal the cannabis industry must be shut down, and the rules that were in place were illegal under international law. From the *Fresh Toast*, we read:

"A secret memo released as part of a recent lawsuit demonstrates how the Trump Administration has quietly blocked marijuana research in the United States. Lawmakers like Joe Biden have lamented not enough marijuana research exists to end federal prohibition, but scientists have just as often lamented tight regulations from the federal government inhibits legitimate research from occurring. Since 1968, scientists pursuing marijuana research have had to obtain their cannabis from a 12-acre farm located at the University of Mississippi. The Obama Administration signed legislation late in 2016 that would expand the number of facilities growing marijuana for research, but the Drug Enforcement Agency hasn't granted any licenses four years later. Thanks to a lawsuit spearheaded by the Scottsdale Research Institute (SRI) and cannabis researcher Sue Sisley, the public now understands why. A 2018 secret memo, released as part of the lawsuit settled, reveals the Trump Administration believes the nearly 50-year-old program in Mississippi has always been illegal. In fact, the Justice Department's Office of Legal Counsel (OLC) suggest the restrictions around marijuana research aren't harsh enough."[26]

---

25 *Lawsuit Forces DEA to Release Secret Internal Memo about Cannabis Research* By Danny Reed -May 1, 2020 MG MAGAZINE
26 *Secret Memo Shows Trump Administration Blocked Marijuana Research For Years*. THE FRESH TOAST. July 14, 2020

According to this article, this Administration believes research on cannabis should be should be *restricted*, to comply with international treaties. Read this memo for yourself, and decide if this is a reasonable interpretation. In my opinion, it is not possible to allow the existence of legal cannabis dispensaries, and keep the regulations outlined in this memo.

The Text of the Memo

This memo instructs the DEA to make changes to comply with UN drug treaties. It gives the DEA has *two* choices: (1) restrict research, license growers, but seize the entire crop after harvest, or (2) prohibit cannabis production altogether. From this memo, titled *Licensing Marijuana Cultivation in Compliance with the Single Convention on Narcotic Drugs,* read:

> "DEA must change policies for single convention. Under the Controlled Substances Act, the Attorney General is authorized to license marijuana cultivation if he determines that it would be "consistent with the public interest and with United States obligations under international treaties, conventions, or protocols in effect on May 1, 1971." 21 U.S.C. § 823(a). Such obligations include those under the Single Convention on Narcotic Drugs ("Single Convention"), Mar. 30, 1961, 18 U.S.T. 1407. As relevant here, the Single Convention requires parties either to prohibit marijuana cultivation altogether or, if they permit cultivation, to establish "a single government agency" to oversee marijuana growers and generally to monopolize the wholesale trade in the marijuana crop. Id. arts. 22, 23(3), 28(1). That single agency must strictly regulate any lawful cultivation of marijuana by, among other things, "purchas[ing] and tak[ing] physical possession of [the] crops as soon as possible, but not later than four months after the end of the harvest." Id. art. 23(2)(d). This opinion considers whether the Drug Enforcement Administration ("DEA"), which exercises the Attorney General's licensing authority, must alter existing licensing practices to comply with the Single Convention. At present, DEA does not purchase or take physical possession of lawfully grown marijuana at any point in the distribution process."[27]

This memo was approved by President Trump's legal council, and circulated by his Administration inside the Drug Enforcement Agency. It instructs them to change the new cannabis policy it announced in 2016:

> "We conclude that DEA must change its current practices and the policy it announced in 2016 to comply with the Single Convention.

27 *Licensing Marijuana Cultivation in Compliance with the Single Convention on Narcotic Drugs.* June 6, 2018

DEA must adopt a framework in which it purchases and takes possession of the entire marijuana crop of each licensee after the crop is harvested. In addition, DEA must generally monopolize the import, export, wholesale trade, and stock maintenance of lawfully grown marijuana. There may well be more than one way to satisfy those obligations under the Single Convention, but the federal government may not license the cultivation of marijuana without complying with the minimum requirements of that agreement."[28]

The DEA announced it would accept more applications from third parties to grown cannabis for research. This was right before President Trump took office. For a year, the delay was based only on pressure from Jeff Sessions, who was taking orders from Donald Trump. While this delay was going on, Trump instructed his legal council to look over current laws, in light of international agreements. Then they released this legal opinion to justify another two years of obstruction.

This stalled over 30 applications. The DEA was told, "current practices" must be changed. As stated, one of these procedures was giving a monopoly to the University of Mississippi to grow all cannabis for research purposes. President Trump's legal decision informs the DEA this practice does not meet the standards of international treaties. Instead, the DEA must "seize" the cannabis crop, and establish a "monopoly."

It is not possible to be this concerned with international treaties, and allow the cannabis industry to legally flourish. It's existence breaks these UN protocols. So, if it *really* is your plan to continue to "allow" states to decide this issue, why be worried about any of these procedures at all? It is not possible to slavishly give such serfdom to these treaties, and not move against the cannabis industry. Why attempt to making these regulations *stricter*— if you are going to continue to allow about a dozen states to break these international rules? The UN has already warned the United States our legal cannabis is illegal[29].

A President who truly cares about the sick would be a leader, and approach Congress to amend the CSA, and send our ambassador to the UN to change these treaties. Instead, the President has gone out of his way to make sure all regulations follow these international protocols. This memo was circulated two years ago, and many of its legal instructions have yet to be implemented. Why? Only one thing stands in the way—the reelection of Donald Trump.

Trump's memo instructs the DEA to control cannabis *as opium*. We read:

"Article 28 of the Single Convention requires that any lawful cultivation of the cannabis plant be subject to the same system of

28 *Ibid*

29 **UN drugs body warns US states and Uruguay over cannabis legalisation**.By Alan Travis. THE GUARDIAN. March 3, 2019

strict controls "as provided in article 23 respecting the control of the opium poppy." Id. art. 28. The cross-referenced provisions in Article 23 provide as follows: 1. A Party that permits the cultivation of the opium poppy for the production of opium shall establish, if it has not already done so, and maintain, one or more government agencies (hereafter in this article referred to as the Agency) to carry out the functions required under this article. 2. Each such Party shall apply the following provisions to the cultivation of the opium poppy for the production of opium and to opium: a. The Agency shall designate the area in which, and the plots of land on which, cultivation of the opium poppy for the purpose of producing opium shall be permitted. b. Only cultivators licensed by the Agency shall be authorized to engage in such cultivation. c. Each license shall specify the extent of the land on which the cultivation is permitted. d. All cultivators of the opium poppy shall be required to deliver their total crops of opium to the Agency. The Agency shall purchase and take physical possession of such crops as soon as possible, but not later than four months after the end of the harvest. e. The agency shall, in respect of opium, have the exclusive right of importing, exporting, wholesale trading and maintaining stocks other than those held by manufacturers of opium alkaloids, medicinal opium, or opium preparations. Parties need not extend this exclusive right to medicinal opium and opium preparations."[30]

So, the President, and his legal team believe *so strongly* in a 60 year-old international treaty, they believe cannabis must be controlled as opium. How could anyone allow the existence of legal dispensaries, and believe this? Furthermore, how can anyone take this position, who believes in medical science? Anyone who believes cannabis is as dangerous as opium, or should be regulated as such, is an idiot. Opiates cause severe addiction, and sometimes death. Cannabis does not.

The President does believe there is *one* difference between cannabis and opium. According to this legal decision, it should be legal to invest in opium, but *illegal* to invest in cannabis stocks.

In the least, this document proves President Trump gladly embraces unscientific UN treaties. It appears he cares more about these agreements, than the votes of the American people. The people have decided to end this prohibition in numerous states. But Donald Trump cares more about obligations to the United Nations.

The legal decisions outlined in this memo should not be ignored. For about a decade, the U.S. Government has looked the other way at legal dispensaries. Two opposing laws have existed side by side. The actions by

30 *Licensing Marijuana Cultivation in Compliance with the Single Convention on Narcotic Drugs.* June 6, 2018

President Trump reveal he plans to change this.

After this memo was released, the DEA again announced they would again accept applications. From Science Magazine, we read:

> "After nearly 4 years of what some researchers saw as foot dragging, the Drug Enforcement Administration (DEA) has announced it will evaluate 37 applications to grow marijuana for medical research and proposed new rules for the prospective growers that outline how the cannabis-growing program would work. "The release of this framework is absolutely monumental and is the biggest, the most meaningful, and material progress made in federal cannabis policy in decades," says George Hodgin, CEO of the Biopharmaceutical Research Company, one of the applicants. "It opens up a path for traditional drug development in the United States," whereby researchers can conduct clinical trials and seek approval from the Food and Drug Administration (FDA) for marijuana-based therapies." [31]

Because the public has been made aware of the medicinal properties of cannabis by many news reports, actions such as these are necessary—*to help the pharmaceutical industry*. Whether by happenstance, or design, that is exactly what these new regulations do. However, this profit is not possible if people continue to have the right to use these substances in their raw form, without a prescription. If everyone can legally grow this plant, their profits are taken away.

In the Federal Register, the DEA explained this change. It was to comply with the Single Convention on Narcotic Drugs. From *Controls To Enhance the Cultivation of Marihuana for Research in the United States,* we read:

> "In 2016, DEA issued a policy statement aimed at expanding the number of manufacturers who could produce marihuana for research purposes... Subsequently, the Department of Justice (DOJ) undertook a review of the CSA, including the provisions requiring consistency with obligations under international treaties such as the Single Convention, and determined that certain changes to its 2016 policy were needed. The pertinent Treaty provisions are found in articles 23 and 28 of the Single Convention, which are summarized below. Additionally, DEA believes that these changes will enhance and improve research with marihuana and facilitate research that could result in the development of marihuana-based medicines approved by the Food and Drug Administration (FDA)." [32]

31 *After 4-year delay, DEA will review dozens of requests to grow marijuana for research* By Greg Miller. SCIENCE. Mar. 30, 2020

32 *Controls To Enhance the Cultivation of Marihuana for Research in the United States.*

These changes were imposed on the DEA by Donald Trump for the same reason the European Union stated that they would not reschedule CBD. These rules are crafted to comply with the *1961 Single Convention.* From the document, we continue to read:

> "Article 23(2) of the Single Convention, made applicable to marijuana cultivation by Article 28, contains five requirements for the supervision, licensing, and distribution of marijuana.[6]
> (a) Designate the areas in which, and the plots of land on which, cultivation of the cannabis plant for the purpose of producing cannabis or cannabis resin shall be permitted.
> (b) Ensure that only cultivators licensed by the agency shall be authorized to engage in such cultivation.
> (c) Ensure that each license shall specify the extent of the land on which the cultivation is permitted.
> (d) Require all cultivators of the cannabis plant to deliver their total crops of cannabis and cannabis resin to the agency and ensure that the agency purchases and takes physical possession of such crops as soon as possible, but not later than four months after the end of the harvest.
> (e) Have the exclusive right of importing, exporting, wholesale trading, and maintaining stocks of cannabis and cannabis resin, except that this exclusive right need not extend to medicinal cannabis, cannabis preparations, or the stocks of cannabis and cannabis resin held by manufacturers of such medicinal cannabis and cannabis preparations.[7]
> DEA already directly performs functions (a), (b), and (c) by virtue of the CSA registration system as applied to manufacturers of marihuana. In order to ensure that DEA complies with the CSA and grants registrations that are consistent with relevant treaty provisions, namely articles 23 and 28 of the Single Convention, DEA proposes to directly perform functions (d) and (e) as well. This proposed rule would amend DEA's regulations so that DEA directly carries out these remaining two functions."

The DEA is supposed to be in charge of all "wholesale trading," according to the Single Convention. Now, there is no way the DEA, or the Trump Administration can allow legal cannabis, and abide by this rule. They can't seize the entire crop, if the vast majority is controlled by dispensaries, regulated by state governments.

After the DEA released these new regulations, the FDA followed suit. The same instructions were given—make new rules to comply with UN agreements. They have released a draft approved by the White House about using "cannabis" in clinical trials. I place "cannabis" in quotes, because it is basically hemp they are talking about regulating.

At the beginning of the document, the FDA tells its employees:

> "This draft guidance, when finalized, will represent the current thinking of the Food and Drug Administration (FDA or Agency) on this topic. It does not establish any rights for any person and is not binding on FDA or the public. You can use an alternative approach if it satisfies the requirements of the applicable statutes and regulations."[33]

So, these new regulations are not *binding* on the FDA, or the public. They are *guidelines* within the agency, approved by the White House. Well, if not binding, how can we trust the government to follow through? Once again, these new rules were written to follow international agreements. The FDA can investigate any cannabinoid as a new drug, *except THC*. Researchers can study any "cannabis"—as long as it tests under 0.3% THC. We read:

> "Other than the specific change to the control status of hemp, scheduling decisions regarding controlled substances were not affected by the 2018 Farm Bill. Activities related to growing and manufacturing cannabis for use as an investigational drug for research must comply with CSA and DEA requirements if the cannabis exceeds the threshold of 0.3 percent delta-9 THC by dry weight. Sponsors and investigators proposing drug development activities involving controlled substances should consult with DEA about the applicable requirements. Sponsors and investigators may find it useful to calculate the level of delta-9 THC in their proposed investigational drug product early in the development process to gain insight into the potential control status of their product."

The FDA is only allowed by law to investigate new drugs, or supplements. This new regulation opens up over 100 cannabinoids, and other substances found in Hemp for medical research. These separately can be investigated in new drug trials, or combinations. After this, these new drugs will be rescheduled as prescriptions, while THC, and CBD remain on "Schedule 1." They will be illegal for you to posess, except in approved prescriptions.

So, President Trump's "expansion"of cannabis research, based on these international treaties, does several things at one time. It purports to open the doors for cannabis research, but THC continues to be restricted. It lays the groundwork for CBD to be fully controlled by the pharmaceutical

---

33 ***Cannabis and Cannabis-Derived Compounds: Quality Considerations for Clinical Research Guidance for Industry, U.S. Department of Health and Human Services Food and Drug Administration Center for Drug Evaluation and Research*** July 2020

industry. Lawyers looked over the precise wording of the UN drug treaties, and interpreted them in a manner that gave CBD and other cannabinoids to this industry.

These drugs will be eventually listed in Schedule 3. At the same time, no drug can be studied with over 0.3% THC, without DEA approval. This continues to give the DEA power to obstruct, or delay. These delays make researching THC too costly, and companies will decide to finance other projects instead.

The investigation of these other cannabinoids might be an attempt to curtail positive news about THC. The discovery of additional substances— that could treat the same conditions—is one way to put the "brakes" on recent reforms. The other way is to present negative information. This Administration appears to be doing both, only the drug companies would control all of these sustances.

These new FDA rules would give pharmaceutical companies a potential windfall of billions of dollars. Even the FDA must contact the DEA, to control the study of THC. We read:

> "We recommend that you consult DEA regarding the control status of cannabis or cannabis-derived materials or products that are under development. We note that intermediates or drug products that contain greater than 0.3 percent delta-9 THC by dry weight, even if the starting materials meet the definition of hemp, may no longer meet the definition of hemp and may be considered a Schedule I controlled substance."

The legalistic lawyers advising President Trump are jumping through hoops to define anything over 0.3 percent THC as a Schedule 1 substance. They hyperinterpret UN treaties exactly as it benefits the drug companies. Other cannabinoids can be studied by the FDA without any barriers:

> "For many years, the National Institute on Drug Abuse (NIDA) Drug Supply Program (DSP)18 87 88 provided the only domestic federally legal source of cannabis for clinical research. Cannabis for 89 the DSP is grown under contract by the University of Mississippi at the National Center for 90 Natural Products Research. However, the changes made by the 2018 Farm Bill allow hemp to 91 serve as a source of cannabis and cannabis-derived compounds for drug development if they do 92 not contain delta-9 THC at more than 0.3 percent by dry weight. This change gives sponsors and 93 investigators of clinical studies new options that do not involve the NIDA DSP."

These new regulations allow sponsors to conduct research on all other cannabinoids under FDA guidance. They must put up money to perform this research. Why invest any money however, if it is legal to go to a dispensary for cannabis, or buy CBD from a store? These new rules were made for a reason. They are worthless, unless your right to access these drugs in their raw form is taken away.

Is This the Only International Agreement the President Cares About?

The National Cannabis industry makes a great point about the Trump Administration, in their response to these new regulations. From their letter, read:

> "Dear DEA: On behalf of the nearly 2,000 members of the National Cannabis Industry Association (NCIA), we appreciate the opportunity to submit comments regarding the Drug Enforcement Administration's (DEA) Request for Information on Controls to Enhance the Cultivation of Marihuana for Research in the United States...To our knowledge, compliance with the Single Convention has never previously been raised as a requirement to obtain a registration. While we believe that the adherence to international treaties is important, DEA's new focus upon the Single Convention is curious to say the least. In recent years, including under the current Administration of President Donald J. Trump, the U.S. has removed itself from multiple international organizations and stopped or limited funding of international organizations. President Trump has not hidden his frustration with international trade groups and security alliances when he has concluded that American national interests required contrary action. Specifically, the Trump Administration has relinquished our responsibilities under numerous international treaties like the Paris Accord, NAFTA, Intermediate Range Nuclear Forces Treaty, Trans-Pacific Partnership, UNESCO, Iran Nuclear Deal, among others. Moreover, the current Administration has regularly railed against international bodies like the United Nations, NATO, World Health Organization, and the UN Human Rights Council that he has concluded were injuring American interests. It is therefore confusing to see how the Administration, which has repeatedly eschewed international treaties over the past four years, is now relying upon an international treaty to justify the transfer of authority over cannabis production for research to law enforcement.[34]

Despite allowing the legal study of these other cannabinoids, THC likely has the greatest therapeutic potential—especially in pain management. From *Pain News Network*, we read:

---

34 *Request for Information on Controls to Enhance the Cultivation of Marijuana for Research in the United States*

"The psychoactive ingredient in marijuana -- tetrahydrocannabinol (THC) – is more effective than cannabidiol (CBD) in treating chronic pain and other medical conditions, according to a new study that challenges the widespread belief that THC is harmful and has limited value in medical cannabis products. Researchers at the University of New Mexico used the Releaf App, a mobile software program, to analyze self-reported data from over 3,300 people who logged their responses in nearly 20,000 user sessions to a variety of cannabis products, including natural dried flower, edibles, tinctures and ointments. Dried flower was the most commonly used product and was generally associated with greater pain relief than other cannabis products, regardless of the amount of THC. "Despite the conventional wisdom, both in the popular press and much of the scientific community that only CBD has medical benefits while THC merely makes one high, our results suggest that THC may be more important than CBD in generating therapeutic benefits," said Jacob Miguel Vigil, PhD, a professor in UNM's Department of Psychology."[35]

According to this study, THC is more effective at treating pain than CBD. Despite the methodology of this study, this is likely true. This means these new rules will keep the opioid market safe. THC has always been it's greatest competitor. If scientists must get permission from the DEA to study extractions over 0.3% THC, research could continue to be delayed for years.

It is possible that President Trump, or some in his cabinet believe the false assumption that THC only gets you high, but therapeutic benefits are found in other cannabinoids. If so, this belief is wrong headed. Most research supports the "entourage effect[36]." THC works together with CBD and other cannabinoids for the greatest benefit. In any case, the new rules work in favor of the pharmaceutical companies, and the genesis of these new rules was a legal decision circulated in a memo President Trump wanted to keep private— because it reveals his true intentions for the industry.

---

35 *Study: THC More Effective Than CBD in Treating Pain*. By Pat Anson. PAIN NEWS NETWORK. February 27, 2019
36 *The Entourage Effect: How CBD and THC Work Together.* By Alan Carter, Pharm.D (written by Raj Chander) HEALTHLINE. December 13, 2019

CHAPTER FOUR:
REEFER MADNESS AT THE TOP

As the memo caused the DEA to delay applications to grow research grade cannabis, people who have the President's ear have provided the White House with selective information. When investigating any issue, the truth cannot be ascertained in the presence of bias. It simply reinforces already held beliefs. If these false beliefs become the basis of policy, laws are created based on lies.

When running for office, the President made numerous pro-cannabis promises. The more you read about his actions however, the more you will understand that he was talking out of both sides of his mouth. While publicly supporting cannabis reforms, he secretly assembled an "anti-cannabis" cabinet. From *Buzz Feed News*, we read:

> "The White House has secretly amassed a committee of federal agencies from across the government to combat public support for marijuana and cast state legalization measures in a negative light, while attempting to portray the drug as a national threat, according to interviews with agency staff and documents obtained by BuzzFeed News. The Marijuana Policy Coordination Committee, as it's named in White House memos and emails, instructed 14 federal agencies and the Drug Enforcement Administration this month to submit "data demonstrating the most significant negative trends" about marijuana and the "threats" it poses to the country... "The prevailing marijuana narrative in the U.S. is partial, one-sided, and inaccurate," says a summary of a July 27 meeting of the White House and nine departments. In a follow-up memo, which provided guidance for responses from federal agencies,

White House officials told department officials, "Departments should provide ... the most significant data demonstrating negative trends, with a statement describing the implications of such trends." As several states have approved laws allowing adults to use and purchase cannabis, critics have contended lax attitudes will promote drug abuse, particularly among youth, and they have pressed for a federal crackdown. The White House at one point said more pot enforcement would be forthcoming, though President Donald Trump has never said he was onboard with that agenda and he announced in June that he "really" supports new bipartisan legislation in Congress that would let state marijuana legalization thrive. However, the committee's hardline agenda and deep bench suggest an extraordinarily far-reaching effort to reverse public attitudes and scrutinize those states. Its reports are to be used in a briefing for Trump "on marijuana threats."[37]

According to this report, the White House assembled this cabinet to *combat* "public support for marijuana." After its existence was made public, Senator Michael Bennet had concerns, and contacted the White House. It responded, acknowledging the report was true. Quoting from the letter, we read:

EXECUTIVE OFFICE OF THE PRESIDENT
OFFICE OF NATIONAL DRUG CONTROL POLICY
Washington, D.C. 20503
September 21, 2018
The Honorable Michael Bennet
United States Senate
261 Russell Senate Office Building
Washington, DC 20510
Dear Senator Bennet:

"Thank you for your recent letter outlining your concerns with the policy coordination process involving marijuana at the Office of National Drug Control Policy (ONDCP). ONDCP sets policies, priorities, and objectives for the nation's drug control programs and ensures that adequate resources are provided to implement them. As such, ONDCP has an obligation to understand the effects drugs have on individuals, public health, and public safety, from a number of different perspectives...The work of ONDCP is based on hard data, science, and evidence from experts in the field. The full range of our counternarcotics efforts are based upon data collected by the Federal Government; the research it performs

---

37 *Inside The Trump Administration's Secret War On Weed*. By Dominic Holden. BUZZFEED NEWS. August 29, 2018

or supports; studies from academic and health experts; and what we learn from law enforcement, healthcare, and public health partners across the country. I assure you that ONDCP seeks all perspectives, positive or negative, when formulating Administration policy. You have my full and firm commitment that ONDCP will be completely objective and dispassionate in collecting all relevant facts and peer-reviewed scientific research on all drugs, including marijuana."[38]

Despite the promise the *Marijuana Policy Coordination Committee* was not approaching this subject with a bias, it apparently is a blatant lie. Everyone in this "anti-cannabis cabinet" submitted "fact sheets" to the President. His administration has claimed executive privilege over these documents, essentially making them secret. From *Reason*, we read:

"The White House Office of National Drug Control Policy (ONDCP) has claimed executive privilege over federal fact sheets that reportedly describe the alleged dangers of marijuana legalization. The agency has thus made the documents secret from the public. In response to a Freedom of Information Act appeal from Reason, the ONDCP asserted that 33 pages of memos sent to its Marijuana Policy Coordination Committee were shielded from release by the presidential communications privilege, under which records prepared or reviewed by the president's close advisers are confidential...Last summer BuzzFeed reported that the ONDCP had a secretive committee on marijuana policy, and that it had ordered more than a dozen federal agencies to submit 2-page fact sheets on the dangers of marijuana legalization. The office solely sought negative information on the drug. The memos instructed 14 agencies and the Drug Enforcement Administration to submit "data demonstrating the most significant negative trends" on the drug and identify issues with state legalization ballot measures, in part to prepare a report for President Donald Trump, who has previously supported states' rights on marijuana."[39]

The White House claims this special cabinet is without bias, yet their recommendations must be kept secret. Why do this, unless their views will hurt Trump's chances for reelection? President Trump knows that 90% of the public supports medical cannabis. If their reports reveal a recommendation to move against the cannabis industry, this is a big problem for his reelection chances.

This group of anti-cannabis activists must have been feeding the

---

38 *The White House Confirms, Yup, It's Been Running A Marijuana Committee.* By Dominic Holden. BUZZFEED. October 21, 2018

39 *Trump White House Claims Executive Privilege Over Agency Memos on Marijuana Legalization.* By C.J. Ciaramella. REASON March 15, 2019

President studies that are of poorer quality, demonstrate bias, or use disputed methods. For example, let's say I want to prove nicotine causes schizophrenia. I know from interviews, that schizophrenics use drugs at a higher rate than the rest of the population—*including nicotine*. So, I go into a mental institution, and interview schizophrenics. I record what I already know, that they use nicotine at a statistically higher rate. Then I publish a study to prove that nicotine causes schizophrenia. Such a study would be seriously flawed. A sample was not used that represented an accurate sample of the population.

Studies with such bias have likely been fed to President Trump, considering some of their claims. The Surgeon General cites some of them his website. President Trump has personally given money to propagate these unsubstantiated claims.

As Governor, Ronald Reagan also believed flawed research, and it caused an important discovery about cannabis to be classified. This study claimed the brains of monkeys were damaged by marijuana use. From the book, the Emperor Wears No Clothes, we read:

"In 1974, California Governor Ronald Reagan was asked about decriminalizing marijuana. After producing the Heath/Tulane University study, the so-called "Great Communicator" told the national press, "The most reliable scientific sources say permanent brain damage is one of the inevitable results of the use of marijuana." (L.A. Times.) And ever since, dead brain cells found in monkeys who were forced to smoke marijuana has been given maximum scare play in federal booklets and government sponsored propaganda literature against pot. In the report, Heath concluded that Rhesus monkeys, smoking the equivalent of only 30 joints a day, began to atrophy and die after 90 days [that's 2700 joints, or an average of 1.25 doobies per hour 24 hours a day, for 90 days!] Heath opened the brains of the dead monkeys, counted the dead brain cells, then took control monkeys who hadn't smokes marijuana, killed them, and counted their dead brain cells. The pot smoking monkeys had enormous amounts of dead brain cells as compared to the "straight" monkeys. Ronald Reagan's pronouncement was probably based on the fact that marijuana smoking was the only difference in the two sets of monkeys. Perhaps Reagan trusted the federal research to be real and correct, therefore reflecting a real health hazard to humans. Perhaps he had other motives. Whatever their reasons, this is what the government ballyhooed to press and PTA, who trusted the government completely. In 1980, Playboy and NORML finally received for the first time -- after six years of requests and suing the government -- an accurate accounting of the research procedures used in the famous report: "The Heath "Voodoo" Research methodology, as reported in Playboy: Rhesus monkeys were strapped into a chair and then strapped into gas masks and given the equivalent of 63 Colombian strength joints in "five minutes, thru the gas masks" losing no smoke. The monkeys were suffocating! When NORML/Playboy hired researchers to examine the reported results against the actual methodology, they laughed. They discovered, almost immediately, that Heath had completely (intentionally? incompetently?) omitted, among other things, the carbon monoxide the monkeys inhaled during these intervals of 63 joints in five minutes...Carbon monoxide is a deadly gas that kills brain cells and is given off by any burning object. All researchers found the marijuana findings in Heath's experiment to be of no value, because carbon monoxide poisoning and other factors involved were totally left out of the report. Three to five minutes of oxygen deprivation causes brain damage..."[40]

Reagan was a good man, yet he was tricked by a "reefer madness" study. It appeared monkeys got brain damage from THC. The details remained unreleased by scientists (as the details of Trump's "Marijuana Policy Coordination Committee" have been kept secret,) for several years. After, the procedures of this study were learned, and it shocked researchers. Monkeys had gas masks strapped on their faces, and forced to constantly smoke joint, after joint, without breathing any oxygen. Carbon monoxide, and lack of oxygen caused the brain damage, not THC.

This one erroneous study caused scientific research into cannabis as a chemotherapeutic agent to be delayed for 10 years. After he became President, Reagan classified 3 studies that revealed THC killed cancer. Few scientists knew they existed, until a freedom of information lawsuit was filed in 1990. Reagan had government agents go to libraries, and colleges, removing pages from publications.

Why would Reagan classify a potential cannabis cure? We cannot know the motives of someone who has passed away. However, it is not unreasonable to assume that his motive was because he *really* believed THC caused brain damage. If cannabis did cause brain damage, this would make it's medicinal use unsuitable for humanitarian reasons.

President Trump could be taking action against cannabis for the same reason. He probably really believes flawed, refutable ideas about this subject. If so, this would make his motives wrongheadedly justified. These beliefs could also excuse reasons that are financially motivated, and non-humanitarian in nature. Many around him reinforce this opinion, such as his new chief of staff. From *Forbes*, we read:

"On Friday, President Donald Trump ousted his acting White House chief of staff, Mick Mulvaney, and replaced him with Rep. Mark Meadows (R-NC). Meadows has consistently opposed efforts to

---

40 From: **The Emperor Wears No Clothes** by Jack Herer

scale back the federal war on marijuana as a member of Congress. Just last month, he was one of 12 GOP lawmakers to send a letter thanking a Senate committee chairman for delaying consideration of a House-passed bill to increase marijuana businesses' access to banks. "We remain opposed to liberalizing drug laws (including around banking), and we see these as some of our areas of greatest concern," Meadows and his colleagues wrote. "We must protect our youth by preventing investment into companies that would prey upon them." [41]

President Trump's chief of staff reveals Trump's opposition to cannabis legalization. They want to prevent cannabis businesses from banking, because they "prey on the youth." Well, do liquor companies "prey on the youth"? I say people in states should begin a petition to "regulate alcohol as cannabis." If cannabis businesses are denied banking, *also deny the alcohol companies* the ability to use the banks. An equal argument can be made that these companies "prey on our youth." But remember, it clearly states in the DEA memo circulated by this Administration, that investments in opiate stocks are fine. This demonstrates either extreme lack of good judgment, or being bought off by drug companies.

As his chief of staff, President Trump's campaign manager stated unequivocally the President is not planning to legalize cannabis. From *Forbes*, we read:

"Asked in a new interview about President Trump's position on changing federal marijuana laws, a top reelection campaign aide said the administration's policy is that cannabis and other currently illegal drugs should remain illegal. "I think what the president is looking at is looking at this from a standpoint of a parent of a young person to make sure that we keep our kids away from drugs," Marc Lotter, director of strategic communications for the Trump 2020 effort, said in an interview with Las Vegas CBS affiliate KLAS-TV. "They need to be kept illegal," he said. "That is the federal policy."[42]

The President's chief of staff publicly stated the President believes the prohibition of cannabis should continue. Trump did *not* rebuke his campaign manager after he said this, neither did he rebuke his chief of staff. This means they are in agreement. His chief of staff stated cannabis prohibition "is the federal policy," and we could add: *"and that's it."* No discussion of whether this policy is just, or moral. Thats the law. Period.

41 *Trump Picks Anti Marijuana Congressman As New Chief Of Staff* By Tom Angell. FORBES Mar 9, 2020

42 *Top Trump Campaign Spokesman: Marijuana Must Be 'Kept Illegal' By Tom Angell.* FORBES February 19, 2020

This position is in direct opposition to the federalism President Trump advocated when he ran for office. The citizens of various States have voted to liberalize cannabis laws, for valid reasons. It takes money away from the black market, which lowers the supply of the drug available to children, frees up police to investigate more serous crimes, frees up the courts of unnecessary cases, and helps lower the overcrowded prison population. In American, one man should not be able to reverse their votes.

Trump Believes Cannabis Lowers IQ

As Reagan believed THC causes brain damage, so President Trump believes another falsehood that might cause him to reject cannabis as a safe pharmaceutical option. From the *Miami Herald*, we read:

> ""The leaked audio also made headlines for Trump calling to "get rid of" then-U.S. ambassador to Ukraine, Marie Yovanovitch, who later testified in U.S. House impeachment hearings. In the same dinner conversation, the topic of marijuana legalization was brought up and Parnas told the president that legal marijuana is "the future, no matter how you look at it." Trump disagreed with the suggestion and mentioned statistics from Colorado, the first state to legalize recreational marijuana. "In Colorado they have more accidents," Trump is heard saying in the leaked audio. "It does cause an IQ problem. You lose IQ points." Audio of the marijuana conversation begins at 45:30 in the video released by Parnas' attorney."[43]

Anti-cannabis activists use the phrase "a permanent drop in IQ" as a pejorative against legalization. It appears the President believes this claim wholeheartedly. Several studies appear to back up this claim, but use methods that could be flawed. For instance, the following study used "self-reports" combined with IQ tests in intervals of 3-6 years. From research published in the *Proceedings of the National Academy of Sciences*, we read:

> "Recent reports show that fewer adolescents believe that regular cannabis use is harmful to health. Concomitantly, adolescents are initiating cannabis use at younger ages, and more adolescents are using cannabis on a daily basis. The purpose of the present study was to test the association between persistent cannabis use and neuropsychological decline and determine whether decline is concentrated among adolescent-onset cannabis users. Participants were members of the Dunedin Study, a prospective study of a birth cohort of 1,037 individuals followed from birth

43 *Marijuana smokers 'lose IQ points,' Trump says in leaked audio. What does science say?* By Mike Stunson. MIAMI HERALD January 28, 2020.

(1972/1973) to age 38 y. Cannabis use was ascertained in interviews at ages 18, 21, 26, 32, and 38 y. Neuropsychological testing was conducted at age 13 y, before initiation of cannabis use, and again at age 38 y, after a pattern of persistent cannabis use had developed. Persistent cannabis use was associated with neuropsychological decline broadly across domains of functioning, even after controlling for years of education. Informants also reported noticing more cognitive problems for persistent cannabis users. Impairment was concentrated among adolescent-onset cannabis users, with more persistent use associated with greater decline. Further, cessation of cannabis use did not fully restore neuropsychological functioning among adolescent-onset cannabis users. Findings are suggestive of a neurotoxic effect of cannabis on the adolescent brain and highlight the importance of prevention and policy efforts targeting adolescents."[44]

Several factors cannot possibly be 100% ascertained by interviews only. These researchers claim they have ruled out other drug, or alcohol abuse, but this is not possible—unless these people were given weekly drug tests. People forget. People lie. People exaggerate. Other factors can also cause an IQ decline unrelated to any kind of substance abuse.

This study makes a claim that anti-cannabis activists repeat over and over again in the media. It was financed by several government agencies from several countries unfriendly to cannabis, including Great Britain, and the United States. Considering the dishonest actions of the government towards cannabis, this alone should make it suspect.

There are studies that purport no decline in IQ. One of them followed two sets of genetically identical twins. From research also published in the *Proceedings of the National Academy of Sciences*, we read:

"Marijuana is one of the most commonly used drugs in the United States, and use during adolescence--when the brain is still developing--has been proposed as a cause of poorer neurocognitive outcome. Nonetheless, research on this topic is scarce and often shows conflicting results, with some studies showing detrimental effects of marijuana use on cognitive functioning and others showing no significant long-term effects. The purpose of the present study was to examine the associations of marijuana use with changes in intellectual performance in two longitudinal studies of adolescent twins (n = 789 and n = 2,277). We used a quasiexperimental approach to adjust for participants' family background characteristics and genetic propensities, helping us to assess the causal nature of

---

44 *Persistent Cannabis Users Show Neuropsychological Decline From Childhood to Midlife Madeline* PROCEEDINGS OF THE NATIONAL ACADEMY OF SCIENCES. PUB MED October 2, 2012

any potential associations. Standardized measures of intelligence were administered at ages 9-12 y, before marijuana involvement, and again at ages 17-20 y. Marijuana use was self-reported at the time of each cognitive assessment as well as during the intervening period. Marijuana users had lower test scores relative to nonusers and showed a significant decline in crystallized intelligence between preadolescence and late adolescence. However, there was no evidence of a dose-response relationship between frequency of use and intelligence quotient (IQ) change. Furthermore, marijuana-using twins failed to show significantly greater IQ decline relative to their abstinent siblings. Evidence from these two samples suggests that observed declines in measured IQ may not be a direct result of marijuana exposure but rather attributable to familial factors that underlie both marijuana initiation and low intellectual attainment."[45]

Two identical twins were studied over several years, one used Cannabis in adolescence, the other abstained. In both cases, the IQ's of these young adults were identical. Another larger study yielded the same results. From the *Journal of Psychopharmacology*, we read:

"There is much debate about the impact of adolescent cannabis use on intellectual and educational outcomes. We investigated associations between adolescent cannabis use and IQ and educational attainment in a sample of 2235 teenagers from the Avon Longitudinal Study of Parents and Children. By the age of 15, 24% reported having tried cannabis at least once. A series of nested linear regressions was employed, adjusted hierarchically by pre-exposure ability and potential confounds (e.g. cigarette and alcohol use, childhood mental-health symptoms and behavioural problems), to test the relationships between cumulative cannabis use and IQ at the age of 15 and educational performance at the age of 16. After full adjustment, those who had used cannabis 50 times did not differ from never-users on either IQ or educational performance. Adjusting for group differences in cigarette smoking dramatically attenuated the associations between cannabis use and both outcomes, and further analyses demonstrated robust associations between cigarette use and educational outcomes, even with cannabis users excluded. These findings suggest that adolescent cannabis use is not associated with IQ or educational performance once adjustment is made for potential confounds, in particular adolescent cigarette use. Modest cannabis use in teenagers may have less cognitive impact than epidemiological

45 *Impact of adolescent marijuana use on intelligence: Results from two longitudinal twin studies.* PROCEEDINGS OF THE NATIONAL ACADEMY OF SCIENCES. PUBMED. January 19, 2016

surveys of older cohorts have previously suggested."[46]

Two studies more accurate debunk a belief held by President Trump about cannabis. Any future actions based on this "fact" would be based on an lie—an "anti-cannabis stereotype." This recent article from *Scientific American* reveals this has yet to be proven. From the Journal of Psychopharmacology, we read:

> "The researchers measured the twins' intelligence between nine and 12 years of age, before any drug use, and did so again between ages 17 and 20. Exactly as in the Dunedin study, marijuana users had lower test scores and showed notable reductions in IQ over time. But in Jackson and Iacono's analysis, marijuana use and IQ were completely uncorrelated, and IQ measures fell equally in both the users and abstainers. Subsequent twin studies, including one performed with U.K. data by the Dunedin team, corroborated these findings of no relationship between marijuana use and a falling IQ. How can we explain these discrepancies? First, young marijuana users are many times more likely to also use alcohol and other illicit drugs. And when epidemiologists factor binge drinking, nicotine and other drug use into their models, marijuana's cognitive effects evaporate. Thus, IQ decline seems more nonspecifically related to general substance use. But this observation doesn't explain why IQ also falls in nonusing twins of cannabis users. Jackson, Iacono and their colleagues noted that at baseline, prior to any substance involvement, future marijuana users in one of the two cohorts they examined already had significantly lower IQ scores. Put another way, cannabis did not drag down their IQ; it was already low." [47]

Despite recent evidence that is contrary to the President's belief, this issue will not be settled until a study is completed in 2027. This will not be long until after Trump leaves office. Evidence up to this point however, is not in his favor. So, to take any actions based on this assertion would be premature.

If President Trump is *really* concerned about a substance that can lower IQ's, he should consider banning alcohol. There is *indisputable* evidence that alcohol causes brain damage, and lowers IQ's. From the website of the *National Institutes of Health*, we read:

> "Difficulty walking, blurred vision, slurred speech, slowed reaction times, impaired memory: Clearly, alcohol affects the brain. Some of these impairments are detectable after only one or two drinks

46 *Are IQ and educational outcomes in teenagers related to their cannabis use?* JOURNAL OF PSYCHOPHARMACOLOGY. SAGE PUBLICATIONS. January 6, 2016

47 *Marijuana May Not Lower Your IQ: Rigorous new studies should be able to settle the matter* By Godfrey Pearlson SCIENTIFIC AMERICAN. May 7, 2020

and quickly resolve when drinking stops. On the other hand, a person who drinks heavily over a long period of time may have brain deficits that persist well after he or she achieves sobriety. Exactly how alcohol affects the brain and the likelihood of reversing the impact of heavy drinking on the brain remain hot topics in alcohol research today. We do know that heavy drinking may have extensive and far–reaching effects on the brain, ranging from simple "slips" in memory to permanent and debilitating conditions that require lifetime custodial care. And even moderate drinking leads to short–term impairment, as shown by extensive research on the impact of drinking on driving."[48]

Alcohol causes brain damage, and a permanent drop in IQ—even among adults. From *Science Daily*, we read:

"Although several studies have shown an association between intelligence and various health-related outcomes, the research on cognitive abilities and alcohol-related problems has been inconsistent. A new study of the association between IQ-test results and drinking, measured as both total intake and pattern of use, has found that a lower IQ is clearly associated with greater and riskier drinking among young adult men, although their poor performance on the IQ-test may also be linked to other disadvantages."[49]

When discussing any drug, you are only scientific if you are consistent. Inconsistency is personal, and almost always flawed. Throughout this book, evidence will be presented that proves *at the least* that nothing can be said bad about cannabis, that is not also true about alcohol, and many other legal drugs. Only in many cases, these substances are far more dangerous than cannabis.

Rallying the Troops

A claim of former Attorney General Sessions has been used against Cannabis many times over the past one hundred and fifty years. This claim has always been debunked by the scientific community. The Attorney General said:

"Experts are telling me there's more violence around marijuana than one would think and there's big money involved."

The problem with his argument: any *real* link between cannabis and violence is because of prohibition. For instance, it is stated that violent crime

---

48 **Alcohol's Damaging Effects on the Brain**. NATIONAL INSTITUTES OF HEALTH. October 2004
49 **A lower IQ has been linked to greater and riskier drinking among young adult men.** SCIENCE DAILY. February 20, 2015

greatly increased in Colorado Springs, after the legalization of recreational cannabis. By making this statement, they are claiming a connection. The problem? Colorado Springs voted against recreational cannabis, and will not allow it. So, this claim fails to recognize many factors, and in the case of Colorado Springs, purposefully manipulates these facts. These claims against cannabis by the government are the "fake news" emerging from "the swamp."

A blanket statement like this is completely unscientific. A similar link has been purported in a recent book, by an author featured many times on Fox News. Alex Berenson has written a book: *"Tell Your Children: The Truth About Marijuana, Mental Illness, and Violence."* This book uses the original title of the movie "Reefer Madness" in a tongue-in-cheek manner, because it purports the same message. It uses inconclusive studies linking cannabis use to schizophrenia, and reports these as fact. The author creates a formula to purport this false premise: (1) Cannabis causes schizophrenia (2) Schizophrenia causes violence and murder, therefore (3) Cannabis causes violence and murder.

This book likely reinforces the beliefs held by many in President Trump's "anti-cannabis cabinet," and uses flawed studies crafted to assume a conclusion. Cannabis as a cause of violence would likely become a key argument of this Administration against legalization, because no one want's to use a pharmaceutical if it causes schizophrenia. The problem is, this is a false premise proven by the prescription drug marinol—synthetic THC—has been on the market for years, with no reports of violence.

Research has been performed with skewed results. Researchers simply go to schizophrenics, interview them about cannabis use, and mark them down as a user if they use it once in a month. These people are not representative of the entire population, neither should occasional cannabis use represent cannabis users.

A group of 75 researchers have criticized the methods of this author:

> "A group of 75 scholars and medical professionals have criticised a controversial new book about the purported dangers of marijuana, calling it an example of "alarmism" designed to stir up public fear "based on a deeply inaccurate misreading of science"."[50]

Another group of physicians, and scientists wrote this about Mr Berenson's claims. In this press release from *Drug Policy.org*, we read:

> "Attributing cause to mere associations. Berenson irresponsibly and dangerously claims a causal link between marijuana use and increases in rates of psychosis and schizophrenia, which have purportedly led to increases in population-level violence. While

---

50 *Popular book on marijuana's apparent dangers is pure alarmism, experts say Doctors and scientists criticize 'flawed pop science' of Tell Your Children – but author Alex Berenson stands by his claims.* The Guardian, Sun 17, 2019

associations between marijuana use and mental illness have been
established, research suggests that the association is complex
and mediated by multiple factors other than marijuana, including
genetics. Similarly, associations between individual characteristics
and violence are multi-factorial. Thus, establishing marijuana as a
causal link to violence at the individual level is both theoretically
and empirically problematic. Further weakening his arguments,
the vast majority of people who use marijuana do not develop
psychosis or schizophrenia, nor do they engage in violence, thus
making Berenson's claims far-reaching and exaggerated."[51]

Some of the quotes used in Berenson's book are from the National
Academies of Sciences. The NAS study only admitted there was a *statistical
relationship* between cannabis use, and schizophrenia. This does not prove
cause, only association. If cannabis relieves these symptoms, this could explain
why this population uses cannabis in a greater percentage. Cause, and treatment
are two possible reasons for this association.
Two of the authors of the National Academies of Sciences objected to
the conclusive manner in which Berenson uses their research. We read:

"The most notable critique comes from one of the researchers who
conducted the study he cites for "arguably the most important
finding of all": a report from the National Academies of Sciences,
Engineering, and Medicine that Berenson claims establishes the
link between psychosis and marijuana. "In response to the recent
@NYTimes editorial on cannabis and as a committee member on
the @theNASEM #cannabis and #cannabinoids report we did NOT
conclude that cannabis causes schizophrenia," pharmacologist
and cannabis researcher Ziva Cooper tweeted in response to an
op-ed by Berenson in The New York Times. Cooper followed this
up with another tweet highlighting two of the study's findings:
an association "between cannabis use and schizophrenia," and
an association "between cannabis use and IMPROVED cognitive
outcomes in individuals with psychotic disorders (not mentioned
in the editorial)."[52]

Mr Berenson's book uses the same tired, refuted argument. A link
between Marijuana and violence has never been established. Instead, drugs
approved by the government can lead to violence. Psychiatric drugs, anti-
psychotics, and anti-depressants, can cause delusions, and violence after sudden

51 *100 Scholars and Clinicians Refute Inaccurate Claims in New Book, Tell Your Children: The
Truth About Marijuana, Mental Illness, and Violence*) DRUG POLICY.ORG. February 15, 2019
52 *What Fear mongering About Pot Tells You About Mainstream Marijuana Coverage. Alex
Berenson's Tell Your Children relies on hyperbole and paranoia to argue against legalization.* THE
NATION. By Katie Way JANUARY 28, 2019

withdrawal. From this study published in *PLOS One*, we read:

> "We identified 1527 cases of violence disproportionally reported for 31 drugs. Primary suspect drugs included varenicline (an aid to smoking cessation), 11 antidepressants, 6 sedative/hypnotics and 3 drugs for attention deficit hyperactivity disorder... Conclusions. Acts of violence towards others are a genuine and serious adverse drug event associated with a relatively small group of drugs. Varenicline, which increases the availability of dopamine, and antidepressants with serotonergic effects were the most strongly and consistently implicated drugs. Prospective studies to evaluate systematically this side effect are needed to establish the incidence, confirm differences among drugs and identify additional common features"[53]

Many drugs currently approved for mental illness can cause violence. The link between cannabis and violence is incorrect, forced, and assumed. It is wrong to interview these people who are on these psychiatric drugs about cannabis use "once in a month," and conclude cannabis caused their violence. They have been given prescriptions that can cause delusions, leading to violent behavior after sudden withdrawal. They attempt to link cannabis to violence using interviews from a subset of the population. This is not accurate.

These two incorrect assumptions—that cannabis causes a drop in IQ, and violence—could become key topics in future anti-cannabis ads, proceeding a shutdown of the industry—in a second Trump Administration.

---

53 *Prescription Drugs Associated with Reports of Violence Towards Others*. PLOS ONE PUBMED. Dec 15 2010

CHAPTER 5:
BLOCKING RESEARCH DELAYED INNOVATION

Regulations written over 40 years ago by Richard Nixon, and the 91st Congress, have delayed research, due to the time, and expense of navigating through the red tape of the Controlled Substance Act. Now we learn the President caused applications to be delayed for three years, while the DEA developed new guidelines. His legal team circulated the memo that stated DEA policies were breaking international laws, and had to be changed.

At the time the Controlled Substance Act was written, Congress appointed a commission to study cannabis—the Shaffer Commission. It recommended that cannabis be decriminalized, based on their investigation. Despite this, Richard Nixon placed cannabis on Schedule 1, and it has remained there ever since. The DEA has refused to remove it from this classification. From *Scientific American*, we read:

"The U.S. Drug Enforcement Administration is announcing today that it will keep marijuana illegal for any purpose (classified as a Schedule I substance under the Controlled Substances Act), but the government will soften rules for marijuana research to make it easier to grow the plant for scientific study. The following article was originally published in the lead-up to this decision. Speculation is growing about the possibility that the U.S. Drug Enforcement Administration (DEA) will review by summer its "Schedule I" designation of marijuana as equal to heroin among the world's most dangerous drugs. Very few Americans know of or understand the DEA's drug-ranking process, and a review of cannabis's history as a Schedule I drug shows that the label is highly controversial and dubious. Disgraced Attorney General

John Mitchell of the Nixon administration placed marijuana in this category in 1972 as part of the ranking or "scheduling" of all drugs under the 1970 Controlled Substances Act. Schedule I drugs are deemed to have no medical use and a high potential for abuse. Cannabis has been there ever since. "As of today, marijuana has never been determined to be medicine," says Russ Baer, staff coordinator in the Office of Congressional and Public Affairs at the DEA. "There's no safe, effective medical use, and a high abuse potential, and it can't be used in medical settings." This determination has come to be insulated by a byzantine, Kafkaesque bureaucratic process now impervious to the opinion of the majority of U.S. doctors—and to a vast body of scientific knowledge—many experts say."[54]

Despite the fact that cannabis is safer than alcohol, the government has regulated it as heroin for more than 40 years. The government is deaf to hundreds of physicians on record stating it has medicinal properties. Furthermore, In order to keep international drug treaties, it is only possible under in US law to move cannabis to Schedule 2. From the *Federal Register*, we read:

"At this time, the known risks of marijuana use have not been shown to be outweighed by specific benefits in well-controlled clinical trials that scientifically evaluate safety and efficacy. The statutory mandate of Title 21 United States Code, Section 812(b) (21 U.S.C. 812(b)) is dispositive. Congress established only one schedule, Schedule I, for drugs of abuse with ''no currently accepted medical use in treatment in the United States'' and ''lack of accepted safety for use . . . under medical supervision.'' 21 U.S.C. 812(b). Although the HHS evaluation and all other relevant data lead to the conclusion that marijuana must remain in schedule I, it should also be noted that, in view of United States obligations under international drug control treaties, marijuana cannot be placed in a schedule less restrictive than schedule II. This is explained in detail in accompanying document titled ''Preliminary Note Regarding Treaty Considerations.'' Accordingly, and as set forth in detail in the accompanying HHS and DEA documents, there is no statutory basis under the CSA for the DEA to grant your predecessors' petition to initiate rulemaking proceedings to reschedule marijuana. The petition is, therefore, hereby denied."[55]

It appears it is your government's position that international treaties

54 *The Science behind the DEA's Long War on Marijuana* By David Downs
SCIENTIFIC AMERICAN April 19, 2016
55 *Denial of Petition To Initiate Proceedings To Reschedule Marijuana*. August 12, 2016

are more important than your access to a natural medication. Schedule 2 drugs must be prescribed with tight controls. According to the DEA in this ruling, cannabis can never be regulated like alcohol. Despite the safety of cannabis, and numerous deaths from alcohol poisoning—booze is okay. Medical science has become secondary to international agreements. Donald Trump, and his legal team have willfully embraced these immutable, unscientific international laws.

40 Years and No Follow Up

Although the FDA, and the DEA continues to deny any medicinal properties in cannabis, another government agency reported the truth about 40 years ago. Ten years of research were performed between 1966 and 1976. This research reported that cannabis could treat numerous conditions. It was published by the National Institute of Drug Abuse in 1977. A document titled, *"Monograph 14: Marihuana Research Findings"*[56] listed many serious, potentially fatal conditions treated by cannabis. Only now—after four decades—are scientists rediscovering these compounds as potential treatments for these diseases. In 1977, scientists knew the following conditions could be treated by cannabis. From *Monograph 14*, we read:

Asthma (Bronchodilation)

"Two lines of research, that of the Vachon group and the work of Tashkin and his collaborators, have clarified a number of questions about the effects of cannabis upon bronchial diameter. Vachon et al. (1973) observed the effects of a single administration of smoked marihuana on normal subjects and on asthmatic patients. They found that airway resistance decreased significantly in the normal group, permitting specific airway conductance and mean expiratory flow rates to increase. In the asthmatics bronchoconstriction was reversed for hours. From subsequent animal work, Vachon et al. (1976a) assume that the bronchodilation that follows -9-THC administration involves the adrenergic system. Recently, Vachon et al. (1976b, 1976c) used a microaerosolized -9-THC spray in 10 asthma This aerosol was found to decrease airway resistance by an average of 16 percent at 90 minutes and increase flow rates without any significant tachycardia or high."

Bronchodilators are a class of drugs that can treat two serious conditions: Asthma and COPD. And now, years later—after countless deaths, researchers are rediscovering this medicinal property. However, the government has discouraged clinical trials. Instead of only being concerned with law enforcement, The DEA must also be the arbiter of scientific research. Not only

---

56 **NIDA.** 1977.

does the cost of regulation dissuade researchers to never apply, the DEA has the power to delay these studies, until they become too costly.

COPD, or Chronic Obstructive Pulmonary Disease is responsible for thousands of deaths each year:

> "COPD refers to a group of diseases that cause airflow blockage and breathing-related problems. COPD affects more than 15 million Americans. More than 140,000 Americans die of COPD each year – that is 1 death every 4 minutes!" [57]

How many people have died of this condition since 1977? In over four decades, there was no serious follow up. Instead of encouraging research by quickly approving applications, the DEA cared more about cannabis prohibition. There is an old saying "add insult to injury." This describes the actions of Donald Trump. It *already* was difficult to navigate the application process in the DEA, but President Trump's legal team has hyper-interpreted international law to make research even harder.

Anticonvulsant

Over the past few years, Cannabis as a treatment for epilepsy has been featured throughout the news. A prescription drug has been made from CBD, Epidiolex. Despite what many believe to be a recent discovery, it was reported in 1977 that cannabis could treat this disease. In *Monograph 14*, we read:

> "Most of the work investigating the anticonvulsant properties of cannabis has been preclinical. The effects of cannabinoids on animal seizures induced by pentylentetrazol (Metrazol), audiogenic or electrical stimulation have been recently examined. Consroe and his associates (Consroe et al., 1973, 1975b; Consroe & Man, 1973) found that -8- and -9-THC blocked all three types of seizures in a dose-related manner. These drugs were qualitatively comparable to diphenylhydantoin (Dilantin). Boggan et al. (1973) also confirmed the effect of -9-THC in mice with induced audiogenic . Dwivedi and Harbison (1975) found that -8- and -9-THC, marihuana extract and uridine protected against pentylentetrazol-induced convulsions in mice. None of these drugs protected against maximal electroshock-induced convulsions. The authors found that their anticonvulsant effects were not additive to diphenylhydantoin, but were additive to phenobarbital."

As other discoveries reported in Monograph 14, there was no follow up. Instead, the government continued to list cannabis among the most dangerous

57 *What is COPD?* CDC.gov

drugs, claiming it had no medicinal properties. How many people have died of epilepsy since 1977? The government restricted cannabis, but approved more dangerous drugs. Many epilepsy drugs cause serious side effects, including nausea, vomiting, weight loss, depression, and many other side effects:

Brivaracetam (Briviact): drowsiness, dizziness, fatigue, nausea and vomiting.

Carbamazepine (Carbatrol or Tegretol): fatigue, vision changes, nausea, dizziness, rash.

Cenobamate (Xcopri): insomnia, dizziness, fatigue, diplopia, and headache

Diazepam (Valium) , lorazepam (Ativan) and similar

Benzodiazepine tranquilizers such as clonazepam (Klonopin): tiredness, unsteady walking, nausea, depression, and loss of appetite. In children, they can cause drooling and hyperactivity.

Eslicarbazepine (Aptiom): dizziness, nausea, headache, vomiting, fatigue, vertigo, ataxia, blurred vision, and tremor.

Ethosuximide (Zarontin): nausea, vomiting, decreased appetite, and weight loss.

Felbamate (Felbatol): decreased appetite, weight loss, inability to sleep, headache, and depression. Although rare, the drug may cause bone marrow or liver failure. Therefore, the use of the drug is limited and patients taking it must have blood cell counts and liver tests regularly during therapy.

Lacosamide (VIMPAT): dizziness, headache, and nausea.

Lamotrigine (Lamictal): dizziness, insomnia, or the potentially deadly Stevens Johnson rash.

Levetiracetam (Keppra): tiredness, weakness, and behavioral changes.

Oxcarbazepine (Oxtellar XR, Trileptal): dizziness, sleepiness, headache, vomiting, double vision , and balance problems.

Perampanel (Fycompa): potential serious events including irritability, aggression, anger, anxiety, paranoia, euphoric mood, agitation, and changes in mental status.

Phenobarbitol: sleepiness or changes in behavior.

Phenytoin (Dilantin): dizziness, fatigue, slurred speech, acne, rash, gum thickening, and increased hair (hirsutism). Over the long term, the drug can cause bone thinning.

Pregabalin (Lyrica): dizziness, sleepiness (somnolence), dry mouth, peripheral edema, blurred vision, weight gain, and difficulty with concentration/attention.

Tiagabine (Gabitril): dizziness, fatigue, weakness, irritability, anxiety, and confusion.

Topiramate (Topamax): sleepiness, dizziness, speech problems, nervousness, memory problems, visions problems, weight loss.

Valproate (Depakote) : dizziness, nausea, vomiting, tremor, hair loss, weight gain, depression in adults, irritability in children, reduced attention, a decrease in thinking speed. Over the long term, the drug can cause bone thinning, swelling of the ankles, irregular menstrual periods. More rare and dangerous effects include hearing loss, liver damage, decreased platelets (clotting cells), and pancreas problems.
Should not be taken if pregnant.
Zonisamide (Zonegran): drowsiness, dizziness, unsteady gait, kidney stones, abdominal discomfort, headache, and rash.[58]

Cannabis prohibition forces epileptics to suffer these side effects in order to stay alive. Instead of respecting people's right to treat their illnesses with a natural substance, the government has kept the safer drug from the people. Some of these side effects are dangerous, including suicidal thoughts. In many cases, doctors must prescribe more than one of these medications. Only after people broke federal law, and discovered the benefits of this plant, were scientists curious, and began to conduct studies. This has led to the development of a prescription medication.

Some forms of epilepsy are rare, and cannot be treated with CBD alone, but require a THC regimen. Some epileptics lucky enough to live in medical cannabis states have discovered this fact. We read:

"Leyland struggled to maintain her ambitious career while grappling with her epileptic symptoms and the awful side effects of the medications. Then one day in 2016 at the urging of a friend she tried a hemp-derived CBD extract. She experienced an immediate, positive shift in her health. "I thought, 'This is what it must be like not to have epilepsy,'" Leyland recalls. "CBD allowed me to feel more normal." For several months, she experimented with different CBD-rich products — both hemp-derived and cannabis-derived, full-spectrum as well as isolate – varying the dosages according to what seemed to work best. Leyland used CBD to wean herself off pharmaceutical meds. But after her initial improvement on a CBD regimen, she still struggled with insomnia, fatigue, and cognitive issues, as well as severe pain from endometriosis and irritable bowel syndrome. Living in New York City, Leyland became a certified medical marijuana patient. In 2018, she went to a state-licensed dispensary in Manhattan and obtained a whole-plant CBD-rich cannabis product that included a healthy percentage of THC. She noticed more pronounced effects right away. "Everything felt sharper," Leyland told Project CBD. "It was like the missing puzzle piece had fallen into place." Chelsea Leyland's experimentation with varying ratios of CBD and THC paid off. Her sleep improved,

58 *Epilepsy Drugs to Treat Seizures.* WEBMD

so did her gut issues. Her seizures went into remission. With THC in the mix, everything settled into a better groove. These days, Leyland says her health is the best it has been in years..”[59]

In some cases, it takes CBD combined with THC to control these seizures. Epileptics should not be made to wait on the government to approve a prescription medication, they should have the right to treat their condition with this plant *now.* Furthermore, because of the outrageous expense of some new prescription drugs, people should not be forced to buy the same substance for triple the price.

Cancer

According to *Monograph 14*, scientists observed in 1977 that cannabis has anti-tumor effects. We read:

“Retardation of Tumor Growth Harris et al. (1976) have reported that mice innoculated with Lewis lung adenocarcinoma showed tumor size reductions ranging from 25-82 percent depending on the dose and duration of treatment with oral 8-THC, -9-THC and cannabinol. No reductions were found with cannabidiol. The effective cannabinoids increased survival time from one-quarter to one-third compared to a 50 percent increase with cyclophosphamide. Friend leukemia virus growth was inhibited by 9-THC, but L1210 murine leukemia was not. In vitro experiments confirmed the inhibition of neoplastic growth in mice, leading the authors to conclude that certain cannabinoids possess antineoplastic properties by virtue of their interference with RNA and DNA synthesis.”

This is the first study that observed THC killing cancer cells. In 1977, NIDA released this document, indicating THC has anti-tumor, anticancer effects. But the government ignored this report, and did not reschedule THC, to make research easier. It is President Trump’s position to keep these restrictions in place, and even make them a little harder. We know this from the DEA memo.

Over one hundred lab, and animal studies have been performed since 1977 that replicated the results of this first study. But only one human trial has be approved. This is the result of blindly following United Nations protocols.

Reports of miraculous recoveries after treating cancer with cannabis oil are found throughout the news, and in PUBMED, in case reports. Of course, not every person has recovered—as with conventional treatments. This is not “fake news” as the Food and Drug Administration claims, but these reports attest to scientific observations made in the lab. From the *Journal of the Association of Basic Medical Sciences*, we read:

59 ***When CBD Isn’t enough to treat Epilepsy.*** By Melinda Misuraca. PROJECT CBD. June 26, 2019

"The plant Cannabis sativa L. has been used as an herbal remedy for centuries and is the most important source of phytocannabinoids. The endocannabinoid system (ECS) consists of receptors, endogenous ligands (endocannabinoids) and metabolizing enzymes, and plays an important role in different physiological and pathological processes. Phytocannabinoids and synthetic cannabinoids can interact with the components of ECS or other cellular pathways and thus affect the development/ progression of diseases, including cancer. In cancer patients, cannabinoids have primarily been used as a part of palliative care to alleviate pain, relieve nausea and stimulate appetite. In addition, numerous cell culture and animal studies showed antitumor effects of cannabinoids in various cancer types. Here we reviewed the literature on anticancer effects of plant-derived and synthetic cannabinoids, to better understand their mechanisms of action and role in cancer treatment. We also reviewed the current legislative updates on the use of cannabinoids for medical and therapeutic purposes, primarily in the EU countries. In vitro and in vivo cancer models show that cannabinoids can effectively modulate tumor growth, however, the antitumor effects appear to be largely dependent on cancer type and drug dose/concentration. Understanding how cannabinoids are able to regulate essential cellular processes involved in tumorigenesis, such as progression through the cell cycle, cell proliferation and cell death, as well as the interactions between cannabinoids and the immune system, are crucial for improving existing and developing new therapeutic approaches for cancer patients. The national legislation of the EU Member States defines the legal boundaries of permissible use of cannabinoids for medical and therapeutic purposes, however, these legislative guidelines may not be aligned with the current scientific knowledge."[60]

Almost no cancer is as deadly as pancreatic cancer. It appears cannabis could also treat this disease. From the *Journal of Pancreatic Cancer*, we read:

"Cannabinoid extracts may have anticancer properties, which can improve cancer treatment outcomes. The aim of this review is to determine the potentially utility of cannabinoids in the treatment of pancreatic cancer. Methods: A literature review focused on the biological effects of cannabinoids in cancer treatment, with a focus on pancreatic cancer, was conducted. In vitro and in vivo studies that investigated the effects of cannabinoids in pancreatic cancer were identified and potential mechanisms of

60 *Cannabinoids in cancer treatment: Therapeutic potential and legislation*. JOURNAL OF THE ASSOCIATION OF BASIC MEDICAL SCIENCES. PUBMED. February 2019

action were assessed. Results: Cannabinol receptors have been identified in pancreatic cancer with several studies showing in vitro antiproliferative and proapoptotic effects. The main active substances found in cannabis plants are cannabidiol (CBD) and tetrahydrocannabinol (THC). There effects are predominately mediated through, but not limited to cannabinoid receptor-1, cannabinoid receptor-2, and G-protein-coupled receptor 55 pathways. In vitro studies consistently demonstrated tumor growth-inhibiting effects with CBD, THC, and synthetic derivatives. Synergistic treatment effects have been shown in two studies with the combination of CBD/synthetic cannabinoid receptor ligands and chemotherapy in xenograft and genetically modified spontaneous pancreatic cancer models. There are, however, no clinical studies to date showing treatment benefits in patients with pancreatic cancer. Conclusions: Cannabinoids may be an effective adjunct for the treatment of pancreatic cancer. Data on the anticancer effectiveness of various cannabinoid formulations, treatment dosing, precise mode of action, and clinical studies are lacking."[61]

Numerous studies like these exist on PUBMED, the online database of the National Library of Medicine, located on the campus of National Institutes of Health (NIH). Some people have researched these studies for themselves, have taken a chance, and beaten the odds. From *the Mirror*, we read:

"George Gannon, 30, received his devastating cancer diagnosis last summer when doctors revealed he had multiple tumours in his brain. After starting chemotherapy, the Hampshire businessman, and his girlfriend began looking at alternatives medicines. In December 2018, George, from Basingstoke, started taking the cannabis oil and by February this year, he decided to quit chemotherapy. Three months later, an MRI scan on his tumours revealed they had actually stopped growing. By August, medics said he was almost completely cancer free."[62]

In my second book on cannabis as a potential cancer cure, I reveal recent discoveries about DNA repair genes, and how they can interfere with any cancer treatment. The cancer killing properties of chemotherapy, or radiation can be neutralized by enzymes produced by these genes. Cannabis oil "down-regulates" these genes, preventing the over-production of these enzymes, and this allows traditional cancer therapies to reach their target. THC itself is a also a

61 *Potential Use of Cannabinoids for the Treatment of Pancreatic Cancer* PUBMED. JOURNAL OF PANCREATIC CANCER. January 25, 2019
62 *Man 'cancer free' after 'cannabis oil helped him beat 12 brain tumours'* By Abigail O'Leary. THE MIRROR. August 27, 2019

cancer killing agent.

As DNA repair genes can interfere with traditional cancer treatments, it appears only *one* of thees gene can disrupt the cancer killing properties of THC. Midkine, or MDK, can neutralize the cancer killing properties of THC. For this reason, not everyone responds to cannabis oil. The complex nature of this issue needs to be studied in depth, in clinical trials.

Recently, the FDA announced: "pot doesn't cure cancer, and stop saying that it does.[63]" The FDA can only truthfully make this statement because clinical trials are almost non-existent. If Trump gets his way—and THC prohibition continues—you will likely have a 50/50 chance of dying of cancer before this issue is fully investigated.

Antibacterial Activity

40 years ago it was revealed that cannabinoids have antibacterial activity. Who knows what could have been learned, if companies did not have to navigate through Schedule 1 regulations! There might be a drug made from cannabis, perhaps combined with other drugs, that could treat or kill the coronavirus. In 1977, these words were written in Monograph 14:

> "Antibacterial Activity In an effort to replicate the work of Kabelik (1957) and Krejci (1958) mentioned earlier, van Klingeren and ten Ham (1976) tested the antibacterial activity of -9-THC and cannabidiol. Broth cultures of staphylococci and streptococci were innoculated with varying concentrations of -9-THC and cannabidiol. They found that both substances were bacteriostatic and bactericidal, but were ineffective against gram negative bacilli. When horse serum was incorporated, the antibacterial effect was greatly reduced, presumably due to protein binding. The utility of these cannabinoids as a topical antibacterial, as suggested by Krejci, seems to have been confirmed on an in vitro basis. Those therapeutic studies that utilize the psychologic effects of marihuana follow."

Of course, the Coronavirus is not a bacteria. Nevertheless, drug resistant bacteria is a current problem that needs a solution. In my last book, I revealed how THC, and CBD are super antibiotics, especially when combined with other drugs. They kill gram-positive bacteria. This could save many lives. Current law however, does not facilitate research.

Sedative-Hypnotic Action

This monograph lists "sedative-hypnotic action" as a medicinal property of cannabis. Sleeping pills kill hundreds of people each year. Cannabis is a safer

---

63 ***Pot Doesn't Cure Cancer and Stop Saying It Does, FDA Says*** by Maggie Fox. November 1, 2017.

alternative. No fatalities have ever been recorded by an overdose, as with prescription drugs. In Monograph 14, we read:

> "Sofia and Knobloch (1973) demonstrated that pretreatment of laboratory animals with -9-THC reduces the dose of barbiturates needed for hypnosis and increases total sleep time. Freemon (1974) confirmed the observation of other investigators that -9-THC, like most hypnosedatives, reduces REM time. However, in contrast to other hypnotics, the abrupt withdrawal of -9-THC after six consecutive nights of usage failed to produce a REM rebound, although mild insomnia was observed."

Because many people suffer from insomnia, newer, more dangerous drugs have been marketed. Ambian, the brand name of Zolpidem, has been linked to violence. From *The Primary Care Companion for CNS Disorders*, we read:

> "Zolpidem is the most commonly prescribed medication for the short-term treatment of insomnia. Adverse reactions include nightmares, confusion, and memory deficits. Reported rare adverse neuropsychiatric reactions include sensory distortions such as hallucinations. Previous research has identified 4 factors that may place a patient at increased risk of zolpidem-associated psychotic or delirious reactions: (1) concomitant use of a selective serotonin reuptake inhibitor (SSRI), (2) female gender, (3) advanced age, and (4) zolpidem doses of 10 mg or higher. In this article, 2 cases are presented in which individuals killed their spouses and claimed total or partial amnesia. Neither individual had a history of aggressive behavior. Both had concomitantly taken 10 mg or more of zolpidem in addition to an SSRI (paroxetine)."[64]

The White house likely embraces the theory that cannabis causes mental illness, which leads to violence. Although untrue, prescriptions such as Ambian are linked to violence, and several deaths. This report indicates that two people did not remember killing their spouses. Because Ambian is in a class of drugs called hypnotics, severe memory loss is possible. Cannabis has never caused memory loss even close to Ambian. Yet the U.S. Government has deemed this drug to be safe, but Cannabis unsafe.

The following class of prescription drugs can cause memory loss:

1. Anti anxiety drugs
2. Cholesterol drugs
3. Anti seizure drugs

64 *Two Cases of Zolpidem-Associated Homicide* THE PRIMARY CARE COMPANION FOR CNS DISORDERS. PUBMED. August 23, 2012

4. Antidepressant drugs
5. Narcotic painkiller
6. Parkinson's drugs
7. Hypertension drugs
8. Sleeping aids
9. Incontinence drugs
10. Antihistamines[65]

Memory loss caused by these drugs is no problem for the government. But any short-term memory loss caused by cannabis is somehow a more serious issue. Intoxication from alcohol also causes memory loss, *even blackouts.*

Analgesia

There have been several decades of opiate abuse and addiction. Many have died. Right now, news stories are reporting that cannabis could be a safer alternative. In 1977, NIDA first reported this in Monograph 14:

"Analgesia One of the earliest folk uses for cannabis was for pain relief. A series of preclinical investigations by Kaymakcalan et al. (1974) tended to confirm this analgesic effect. After having received intravenous administrations of 1 mg/kg -9-THC, dogs received electric stimulation through an implanted dental electrode. The cannabinoid produced a definite analgesic effect, as shown by a fourfold increase in pain thresholds. Tolerance to analgesia, sedation and ataxia occurred in eight days. In another study, -9-THC produced pain reduction in mice and rats as measured by tail flick and writhing tests, and in rabbits receiving sciatic nerve stimulation. The analgesia produced with the doses used was equivalent to morphine analgesia -- in fact, in rats, a cross tolerance between -9-THC and morphine was found. An earlier study (Parker & Dubas, 1973) measured the effect of -9-THC on rats with electrodes implanted in aversive brain sites. A nondose related elevation of the pain threshold and an attenuation of the escape response were also recorded."

How many lives could have been saved, if cannabis were a legal option for pain? States that legalized cannabis witnessed a sharp decline in opiate use. In *Scientific American*, we read:

"As more states legalize medical and recreational marijuana, doctors may be replacing opioid prescriptions with suggestions to visit a local marijuana dispensary. Two papers published Monday

---

65 ***AARP. Caution! These 10 Drugs Can Cause Memory Loss***. by Dr. Armon B. Neel, Jr., February 9, 2016

in JAMA Internal Medicine analyzing more than five years of Medicare Part D and Medicaid prescription data found that after states legalized weed, the number of opioid prescriptions and the daily dose of opioids went way down. That indicates that some people may be shifting away from prescription drugs to cannabis, though the studies can't say whether this substitution is actually happening or if patients or doctors are the driving force. "In this time when we are so concerned—rightly so—about opiate misuse and abuse and the mortality that's occurring, we need to be clear-eyed and use evidence to drive our policies," said W. David Bradford, an economist at the University of Georgia and an author of one of the studies. "If you're interested in giving people options for pain management that don't bring the particular risks that opiates do, states should contemplate turning on dispensary-based cannabis policies.""[66]

Because cannabis is not a legal option in all 50 States, not everyone can access this safer medication. We have the Federal Government to thank for that. Opiates are legal, cannabis is not. Opiates kill by overdose, cannabis does not. President Trump's legal team supports legal investments in opiate stocks, but not cannabis. Hundreds may have died because politicians refuse to reform these laws.

Antidepressant

As previously stated, antidepressants can be deadly. Every year, many people die of overdose, or experience severe mental issues upon sudden withdrawal. In 1977, researchers discovered cannabis has antidepressant properties. We read:

"Since marihuana tends to elevate mood, it follows that an evaluation of its antidepressant potential would be sought. Kotin et al. (1973) administered 0.3 mg/kg of -9-THC or a matching placebo twice daily to eight patients who required hospitalization for their affective disorder. The patients were all considered moderately or severely depressed. Treatment lasted a week, with placebos substituted for the active drug thereafter. No evidence of a significant affectual change could be demonstrated. In chronic depressive states, a longer duration of drug administration is sometimes needed before improvement is noted. A group at the Medical College of Virginia (Regelson et al., 1976) performed a double blind study with cancer patients receiving chemotherapy. An initial starting dose of 0.1 mg/kg t.i.d. was used. The dosage

66 *Where Marijuana Is Legal, Opioid Prescriptions Fall.* By Kate Sheridan, SCIENTIFIC AMERICAN. April 2, 2018

was raised only if previous doses were welltolerated. On a battery of personality tests and mood scales, the -9-THC acted as a mood elevator and tranquilizer producing significant improvement on two of three Zung depression scales. Cognitive functioning was unimpaired and appetite enhancement and retardation of weight loss were noted from clinical records. The need for narcotics was decreased, and patients had the impression that some pain relief resulted."

NIDA reported cannabis could treat depression in 1977, but our government refused to change the law. They kept cannabis on Schedule 1, which only gave people the option to access drugs far more dangerous, with serious side effects. In Great Britain, one study has linked antidepressants to *28 murders.* From *the Sun*, we read:

> "The common antidepressants are considered safe for the vast majority of patients. But there have been reports linking them to psychosis, violence and in extreme cases, murder. Experts warn that in rare circumstances the pills can trigger dangerous mood swings. Using Freedom of Information laws, BBC Panorama found 28 cases where the drugs have been implicated in a murder and 32 where users complained of murderous thoughts."[67]

People have died because the government thinks it knows better. As Ronald Reagan so adequately stated, "Government is not the solution to our problem, government *is* the problem." His words certainly ring true about cannabis prohibition. The CSA is supposed to be a law that protects, but instead it harms. A safer drug has been kept from the people, while the more dangerous drugs have been approved. Several mass murders have happened after people withdraw from these medications. Only now scientists are "rediscovering" cannabis as a safer option. From *Pain News Network*, we read:

> "Consuming dried cannabis flowers significantly reduces symptoms of depression and works much faster than pharmaceutical antidepressants, according to a new study of over 1,800 cannabis consumers. The study findings, published in the Yale Journal of Biology and Medicine, is the latest research derived from the Releaf App, a free mobile software program that collects self-reported, real-time information from people on their use of cannabis and its effect on chronic pain, depression and over two dozen other medical conditions. This particular study excluded the use of cannabis edibles, lotions and oils, and focused solely on cannabis buds that were smoked or inhaled through a

<hr>

67 ***Common antidepressants 'linked to at least 28 murders in the UK', investigation reveals.*** By Nick McDermott, THE SUN. July 26, 2017

vaporizer. Over 95% of participants in the study reported a decline in depression within hours of ingesting cannabis, with an average reduction in symptom intensity of nearly 4 points, based on a numerical zero to 10 depression scale. "[68]

Withdraw from cannabis is mild, causing only sleep disturbances, and slight irritability for a few days. There is no "antidepressant rebound." This "rebound" can cause mania, suicide, violence, and murders.

Treatment of Alcohol and Drug Dependence

For years, politicians claimed Cannabis was a "gateway drug." Yet in 1977, Monograph 14 reported the exact opposite:

"Rosenberg (1976) has studied the response of a group of alcoholics and normal volunteers to marihuana cigarettes (0.4 gm/50 lb. body weight) and to alcohol (2 ml vodka/kg.).This investigator found that sober alcoholics tended to be less responsive to stresses (mental arithmetic and talking to a videocamera) and were more likely to withdraw from a stress situation than the normals. Alcoholics became more angry and depressed after alcohol ingestion as measured by mood scales. Marihuana produced a more positive mood state and did not interfere with the arousal reaction, although it greatly increased heart rate and produced an acute paranoid or confusional state in 3 of the 27 subjects. This investigator also found that disulfiram (Antabuse) and marihuana could be given safely together in the treatment of alcoholism."

The U.S. government had data that cannabis could treat drug addiction, but instead kept it illegal, claiming the opposite. With legal access, people could have used cannabis to treat serious addictions. Cannabis only leads to other drugs *because it is illegal*. People go to friends, and buy cannabis from the black market. One day their friends might diversify, and begin selling cocaine, crack, heroin, and other dangerous drugs. Thus people are exposed to other drugs because of cannabis prohibition. Prohibition creates the drug pusher, a term not used much anymore by the government—because they want to blame cannabis.
Monograph 14 concludes with this statement:

"The further study of the cannabinoids for various therapeutic applications seems worthwhile. A large number of synthetic cannabinoids have begun to appear which do not have some of the disadvantages intrinsic in the naturally occurring ones. Therapeutic

____

68 Study Finds Cannabis Effective for Treating Depression. By Pat Anson. PAIN NEWS NETWORK. July 03, 2020.

efficacy could be enhanced by certain molecular manipulations. Thus, it is likely that if any cannabinoid ever achieves clinical acceptance, it will be a synthetic. The cannabinoid configuration would be important to human therapeutics because: 1) there is a wide safety margin between effective and lethal doses, and 2) in certain instances, the mechanism of action appears to differ from the standard medications now employed."

The physician who wrote these words—way back in 1977—concluded cannabis is a safer alternative to many prescription medications. President Trump has demonstrated by his actions he does not believe this. He has blocked cannabis research, and is out of step with the American people on this issue.

Cannabis Might Treat COVID-19

The greatest crisis of the Trump presidency is this current pandemic. The country was unprepared when this crisis hit, despite any mistakes the President may, or may not have made. Yet, what could we have learned, if cannabis were not listed in Schedule 1, all of those years? As stated, scientists knew in 1977 that THC, and CBD had antibacterial properties. The laws remained restricted, so no investigation was made.

Without restrictions on cannabinoid science, we might have an approved cannabis based drug to treat the "cytokine storm" caused by COVID-19. Lives might have been saved, and the economy never shut down. It was reported recently that cannabinoids might prevent the Coronavirus from binding to human cells. From the *Atlanta Journal-Constitution*, we read:

> "Researchers at the University of Lethbridge recently released results from a study that shows the benefits of CBD as an aid in blocking the cells that enter the body from the novel coronavirus. The study, published in peer journal Preprints, was conducted by the scientists in April, and the results were released in a non-peer-reviewed, preclinical study titled "In Search of Preventative Strategies: Novel Anti-Inflammatory High CBD Cannabis Sativa Extracts Modulate ACE2 Expression in COVID-19 Gateway Tissues" earlier this month, according to a release from pharmaceutical research company Pathway RX. [69]

We also read this from the *Calgary Herald*:

> "Cannabis extracts are showing potential in making people more resistant to the novel coronavirus, says an Alberta researcher leading a study. After sifting through 400 cannabis strains,

69 ***Canadian Study finds that Enzymes in Cannabis could treat COVID-19.*** By Stephanie Toone. THE ATLANTA JOURNAL-CONSTITUTION.

researchers at the University of Lethbridge are concentrating on about a dozen that show promising results in ensuring less fertile ground for the potentially lethal virus to take root, said biological scientist Dr. Igor Kovalchuk. "A number of them have reduced the number of these (virus) receptors by 73 per cent, the chance of it getting in is much lower," said Kovalchuk. "If they can reduce the number of receptors, there's much less chance of getting infected. The study sought ways to hinder the highly contagious virus from finding a host in the lungs, intestines, and oral cavity."[70]

In *"CBD and the Cytokine Storm,"* I quoted research first performed 20 years ago that proved cannabinoids are immunomodulators, and can contradict the "cytokine storm" in lab animals. This over-active immune response causes the fatal pneumonia associated with COVID-19, and both CBD, and THC contradict it. Since this discovery, people continued to die of pneumonia, while this potential treatment was ignored by the government.

Israel however, appears to have laws more conducive to research. They are testing CBD on COVID-19 right now. From *the Ledger,* we read:

"(JNS) The Israel-based biotech company Stero Biotechs has started a small-scale clinical trial at Rabin Medical Center's Golda Hasharon Campus in Petach Tikvah on the effects of a steroid-Cannabidiol (CBD) treatment on hospitalized COVID-19 patients. "Steroid treatment is usually the rst or second line of treatment for hospitalized patients. CBD enhances the therapeutic effect of steroid treatment and treats the bio-mechanism affected by the virus," the company said in a press release announcing the clinical trial. "The initial study will evaluate the tolerability, safety and ecacy of the CBD treatment for hospitalized patients with COVID-19 Infections." Ten patients will be in the clinical trial; the treatment cycle will be for a few weeks with a follow-up period of the same length."[71]

Monograph 14 stated that THC, and CBD have antiviral properties. 20 years ago, studies in lab animals indicated both THC, and CBD could stop lung infections caused by the same immune response as COVID-19. Only now are researchers rediscovering this effect:

"Acute Respiratory Distress Syndrome (ARDS) is a life-threatening complication that can ensue following Staphylococcus aureus infection. The enterotoxin produced by these bacteria (SEB)

70 *Cannabis shows promise blocking coronavirus infection: Alberta researcher*. By Bill Kaufman. CALGARY HEROLD. May 7, 2020

71 *Israeli biotech company starts clinical trials of CBD-steroid treatment for virus* LEDGER ONLINE. May 5, 2020

acts as a superantigen thereby activating a large proportion of T cells leading to cytokine storm and severe lung injury. Δ9Tetrahydrocannabinol (THC), a psychoactive ingredient found in Cannabis sativa, has been shown to act as a potent anti-inflammatory agent. In the current study, we investigated the effect of THC treatment on SEB-induced ARDS in mice. While exposure to SEB resulted in acute mortality, treatment with THC led to 100% survival of mice." [72]

In one study, CBD worked better than steroids to treat COVID-19:

"In the last few months, researchers have been looking at whether cannabis, or it's many chemical compounds, might help to fight this deadly effect by bringing down inflammation. Recently, we've seen positive results from studies suggesting that CBD, a compound in cannabis, may help fight these cytokine storms. Now early results from an ongoing Israeli study are adding to the chorus of researchers suggesting that cannabis' ingredients could be a game changing treatment in the fight against Covid-19. But this study says that terpenes, compounds that provide the aroma and flavor in cannabis and many other plants, may lead to even better results than CBD alone, and might outperform conventional treatments like corticosteroids. Reports from the study show that a combination of CBD with terpenes was 3 times more effective at inhibiting cytokine activity than dexamethasone, a corticosteroid which a recent study found to be an effective treatment for Covid-19 cytokine storms."[73]

Clinical studies into cannabis as a treatment for this disease were performed in other countries, with their approval. Current laws embraced by Donald Trump allow foreign governments to lead in cannabinoid research. Yet, by simply analyzing the data, researchers from several American universities have confirmed this possibility:

"Coronavirus disease-2019 (COVID-19), caused by Severe Acute Respiratory Syndrome coronoavirus-2 (SARS-CoV2) has emerged as a global pandemic, which was first reported in Wuhan, China. Recent reports have suggested that acute infection is associated with a cytokine superstorm, which contributes to the symptoms of fever, cough, muscle pain and in severe cases bilateral interstitial

72 *Administration of Δ9-Tetrahydrocannabinol (THC) Post-Staphylococcal Enterotoxin B Exposure Protects Mice From Acute Respiratory Distress Syndrome and Toxicity*. PUBMED. June 16, 2020
73 *New Research Suggests Terpenes And CBD Work 2X's Better For Covid-19 Inflammation Than Corticosteroid*. By Emily Earlinbaugh. FORBES. July 21, 2020

pneumonia characterized by ground glass opacity and focal chest infiltrates that can be visualized on computerized tomography scans (Rothan and Byrareddy, 2020). Currently, there are no effective antiviral drugs or vaccines against SARS-CoV2. In the recent issue of BBI, Zhang et al. (Zhang et al., 2020) thoroughly summarized the current status of potential therapeutic strategies for COVID-19. One of them, anti-IL6 receptor (Tocilizumab) antibody, resulted in clearance of lung consolidation and recovery in 90% of the 21 treated patients (Fu et al., 2020). Although promising, it has also produced adverse effects like pancreatitis and hypertriglyceridemia (Morrison et al., 2020), which make it imperative to explore effective alternative anti-inflammatory strategies. Here, we intend to highlight the potential effects of cannabinoids, in particular, the non-psychotropic cannabidiol (CBD), that has shown beneficial anti-inflammatory effects in pre-clinical models of various chronic inflammatory diseases and is FDA approved for seizure reduction in children with intractable epilepsy (Nichols and Kaplan, 2020). Like Δ9-tetrahydrocannabinol (Δ9-THC), the most well-studied cannabinoid, CBD decreased lung inflammation in a murine model of acute lung injury potentially through the inhibition of proinflammatory cytokine production by immune cells and suppressing exuberant immune responses (Ribeiro et al., 2015). CBD can inhibit the production of proinflammatory cytokines like interleukin (IL)-2, IL-6, IL-1α and β, interferon gamma, inducible protein-10, monocyte chemoattractant protein-1, macrophage inflammatory protein-1α, and tumor necrosis factor-α (Nichols and Kaplan, 2020) (Fig. 1) that have been associated with SARS-CoV2 induced multi-organ pathology and mortality. In a murine model of chronic asthma, CBD reduced proinflammatory cytokine production, airway inflammation and fibrosis (Vuolo et al., 2019). Moreover, CBD can effectively inhibit the JAK-STAT pathway including the production and action of type I interferons without leading to addiction, alterations in heart rate or blood pressure and adverse effects on the gastrointestinal tract and cognition (Nichols and Kaplan, 2020). In simian immunodeficiency virus (SIV)-infected rhesus macaques (RMs), we reported THC mediated attenuation of IFN stimulated gene expression in the intestine (Kumar et al., 2019). Similar to CBD, chronic THC administration blocked inflammation induced fibrosis in lymph nodes of chronically SIV-infected RMs (Kumar et al., 2019). Unlike THC, CBD has a high margin of safety and is well tolerated pharmacologically even after treatments of up to 1500 mg/day for two weeks in both animals and humans (Nichols and Kaplan, 2020), which suggests its feasibility to reduce SARS-CoV2 induced lung inflammation/pathology and disease severity."[74]

Animal studies confirmed that THC, and CBD could treat the "cytokine storm" over 20 years ago. But what happened? The schedule 1 status of cannabis made it too costly, and time consuming for any company to finance research. They understand the delays, and the opinion of the government on this issue. They have heard what other researchers have gone through. So, a potential treatment for this current pandemic was never explored. You can thank cannabis prohibition for this—and President Trump would continue it.

Treats MRSA

As revealed in Monograph 14, THC, and CBD are antibacterial agents. MRSA, the flesh eating virus, kills more people than AIDS every year. If someone is infected with a antibiotic resistant strain, the flesh rots off of their body. Researchers discovered substances in Cannabis kill this bacteria. *From Brain, Behavior, and Immunity*, we read:

> "Study Shows Cannabinoids May Be Useful Against Drug-Resistant Staph Infections By Caroline Wilbert Chemicals in marijuana may be useful in fighting MRSA, a kind of staph bacterium that is resistant to certain antibiotics. Researchers in Italy and the U.K. tested five major marijuana chemicals called cannabinoids on different stras of MRSA ... All five showed germ-killing activity against the MRSA strains in lab tests. Some synthetic cannabinoids also showed germ-killing capability. The scientists note the cannabinoids kill bacteria in a different way than traditional antibiotics, meaning they might be able to bypass bacterial resistance. At least two of the cannabinoids don't have mood-altering effects, so there could be a way to use these substances without creating the high of marijuana."[75]

Five separate cannabinoids in Cannabis has been found to kill the MRSA virus in the lab. Yet, people continue to die from this disease. A gap of almost 40 years has occurred, before any serious investigations. Companies simply did not want to deal with regulations of a substance so tightly controlled. This bureaucratic "red tape" has been *thickened* during the Trump Administration.

THC is a Possible Treatment for Alzheimer's

Alzheimer's disease causes confusion, memory loss, and death. The United States government has a patent on THC, and CBD, as neuroprotectant

---

74 *SARS-CoV2 induced respiratory distress: Can cannabinoids be added to anti-viral therapies to reduce lung inflammation?* BRAIN, BEHAVIOR, AND IMMUNITY. PUBMED. July, 2020

75 *Chemicals in Marijuana May Fight MRSA*. WEBMD. September 4, 2008

agents. They are potential treatments for brain damage, and Alzheimer's disease. From the *Denver Post*, we read:

> "Patent No. 6,630,507: Why the U.S. government holds a patent on cannabis Patent No. 6,630,507. In the case of No. 6,630,507, the researchers discovered that nonpsychoactive compounds in cannabis may have antioxidant properties that could be beneficial in the treatment of certain neurological diseases, she said...The patent doesn't prove the chemical compound is effective in the stated treatment, Rohrbaugh said. The compound would have to be purified, synthesized in a lab setting, subjected to extensive testing in animals and humans, and ultimately require U.S. Food and Drug Administration approval to show that it's safe and effective for the intended purpose."[76]

Thousands of people suffer, and die from Alzheimer's every year. Before cannabis is used as a treatment however, it would have to be "subjected to extensive testing in animals and humans, and ultimately require U.S. Food and Drug Administration approval..." Because the U.S. Government has refused to reschedule Cannabis, no companies have attempted to investigate this for years. Nevertheless, researchers have recently rediscovered this medicinal property:

> "An active compound in marijuana called tetrahydrocannabinol (THC) has been found to promote the removal of toxic clumps of amyloid beta protein in the brain, which are thought to kickstart the progression of Alzheimer's disease. The finding supports the results of previous studies that found evidence of the protective effects of cannabinoids, including THC, on patients with neurodegenerative disease. "Although other studies have offered evidence that cannabinoids might be neuroprotective against the symptoms of Alzheimer's, we believe our study is the first to demonstrate that cannabinoids affect both inflammation and amyloid beta accumulation in nerve cells," says one of the team, David Schubert from the Salk Institute for Biological Studies in California. Schubert and his colleagues tested the effects of THC on human neurons grown in the lab that mimic the effects of Alzheimer's disease."[77]

It appears this neuroprotective ability of Cannabis also protects against age related memory loss. From *Discover Magazine*, we read:

---

76 ***Patent No. 6,630,507: Why the U.S. government holds a patent on cannabis plant compounds*** By Alicia Wallace. DENVER POST. October 2, 2016
77 ***Marijuana Compound Removes Toxic Alzheimer's Protein From The Brain*** May 26, 2018. SCIENCE ALERT

"A longtime U.S. National Institutes of Health (NIH) researcher who is now one of Germany's most respected neuroscientists, Zimmer has been on a long journey to answer a question that few researchers had thought to ask: Is it possible that weed, long seen as the stuff of slackers, might actually contain the secret to sharpening the aging brain? His findings have suggested that may be the case. As the data continues to stream in, some in the lab have begun quietly encouraging their aging parents to toke away, laws be damned. "I sent my mother recipes for baking pot cookies," says one researcher in Zimmer's lab, who asked not to be identied because it's still illegal in the mother's country. In 2005, Zimmer's research was the first to provide convincing evidence that synthetic THC seems to slow age-related brain degeneration. His results since then, combined with a general renaissance in cannabis research that parallels the growing popular and political acceptance of weed, has added more weight to that theory and spurred the interest of labs around the world. Until recently, most of the research has been conducted on mice. But newer research conducted at Johns Hopkins University, Harvard Medical School-afliated McLean Hospital, and the University of Colorado, among other places, has already suggested that at least some of the benefits of THC — the component primarily responsible for marijuana's psychoactive effects — accrue in humans' aging brains. Taken together, this progress has set off a worldwide race to nail down solid proof that, as unlikely as it may sound, pot works in humans to slow, and possibly reverse, Alzheimer's and other forms of dementia."[78]

In studies, THC caused the intellect of younger mice to be slightly dulled while stoned; but the older mice were more cognizant, and mentally agile. It made the older mice *slightly* smarter. This lab experiment confirms the validity of the U.S. Patent, but has had little clinical investigation because of laws *embraced by the Trump Administration*.

How many people could be harmed by your vote?

The sick need access to cannabis now. It takes an average of 15 years before a new drug is approved, and marketed. Many cannot wait. Some of these conditions can kill. This chart lists some of the conditions cannabis could potentially treat, and also how many years passed before investigation:

---

78 *The Experiments Revealing How Marijuana Could Treat Dementia.* By David H. Freedman. DISCOVER MAGAZINE. February 7, 2020

Year First Reported	Condition	Result (as June, 2020)
1977	Bronchodilation (asthma)	Few human studies, no medications tested
1977	Anticonvulsant (epilepsy)	No human studies, until recent cannabis reforms
1977	Retardation of Tumor Growth (cancer)	One limited clinical trial in 2018, with promising results
1977	Antibacterial Activity (gram positive antibiotic)	No human studies, until the Coronavirus pandemic
1977	Sedative-Hypnotic Action (sleep aid)	No human studies, until recent cannabis reforms
1977	Analgesia (pain)	No human studies, until recent cannabis reforms
1977	Treatment of Alcohol and Drug Dependence	No human studies, until recent state financed studies, due to cannabis reforms
1977	Antidepressant.	One study in 2020; only self reporting
1977	Anti-nauseant, Antiemetic and Appetite Enhancer	Synthetic cannabinoid drug Marinol tested, and approved in 1985
1991	"Cykotine Storm"	No human studies, only lab animals, until Coronavirus outbreak
1999 US Patent US6630507B1	Alzheimer's	No human studies, until recent cannabis reforms
1999 US Patent US6630507B1	Head Injuries	No human studies, until recent cannabis reforms
1999 US Patent US6630507B1	Stroke	No human studies, until recent cannabis reforms
2008	MRSA	Pre-clinical studies after cannabis reforms
2019	Age related memory	Pre-clinical studies after cannabis reforms
2020	Coronavirus (prevention of ACE receptor binding)	2020: Studies ongoing in Canada

| 2020 | COVID-19 (Cytokine Storm) | 2020: Studies ongoing in Israel |

The status quo has caused research into these conditions to be delayed for years. Already, lives have been lost to some of these illnesses. The existence of the DEA memo, the new cannabis rules, and the "anti-cannabis" cabinet— all indicate this Administration supports these bad laws, and would even make them worse. So, if you rely on cannabis to treat any of these illnesses, *you will be voting against your own life, and health, if you vote for Donald Trump.*

CHAPTER 6:
TRUMP'S DONATION AGAINST CANNABIS

In this chapter, I will try attempt to answer every objection to legalization given by this Administration through the Surgeon General. President Trump personally financed warnings about cannabis, posted on the government website. Since these arguments would be used prior to an industry wide shutdown, I will present studies that address these issues, and I will also attempt to anticipate, and answer additional arguments that could be used.

Instead of keeping his campaign promise to support medical cannabis, his legal team has reinterpreted current regulations to impose *stricter* rules on cannabis. Trump informed the DEA, it must change it's practices, to comply with international laws. It is unimaginable these new procedures would not be fully enforced, if President Trump is reelected.

Looking ahead towards this future enforcement, President Trump has donated $100,000 of his salary to finance these misleading claims:

> "Officials with the Trump administration spoke out against cannabis this week. First, the United States Surgeon General issued an advisory warning about the harms of cannabis consumption. "The legalization movement may be impacting youth perception of harm from marijuana," the advisory stated. The advisory was largely directed at pregnant women and adolescents and its publication will be partially funded by a $100,000 donation from President Donald Trump's salary. Later in the day Trump cabinet official Alex Azar (Health and Human Services) was on Fox Business promoting the advisory, but in the process, inadvertently made the case for a regulated cannabis industry when he himself pointed out that the unregulated cannabis industry doesn't have consumer labels, which would obviously help with addressing

concerns about public health education." [79]

The statement that "no amount of cannabis is safe," is ludicrous, incorrect, and is laughable considering the dangers of numerous prescription drugs, all approved by the FDA. Based on all of Trump's actions, it appears this donation is merely one step towards softening public opinion before the feds shut down the cannabis industry. Of course, other anti-cannabis groups are likely waiting to contribute to a greater ad campaign after a shutdown begins.

Trump's donation is merely symbolic, but is a one step towards the goal of the "Marijuana Policy Coordination Committee." Public support must be changed. Nevertheless, the *content* of the message he financed should be scrutinized, and it will in this chapter. He knows public opinion must be changed, or his actions would be despised. However, if he believes he is doing right, *he will not care*, but will "dig in," and move forward. This is the dangerous side of his personality.

The Surgeon General's Warning

The office of the Surgeon General has posted Trump's "anti-cannabis" message online. In these words, we can understand what kind of commercials the government will likely run sometime after his reelection. Here is the message posted on the website, analyzed with studies considered to be more accurate, because of the methods used. In the beginning of the Surgeon General's warning, we read:

> *"Marijuana, or cannabis, is the most commonly used illicit drug in the United States. It acts by binding to cannabinoid receptors in the brain to produce a variety of effects, including euphoria, intoxication, and memory and motor impairments. These same cannabinoid receptors are also critical for brain development. They are part of the endocannabinoid system, which impacts the formation of brain circuits important for decision making, mood and responding to stress.*
>
> *Marijuana and its related products are widely available in multiple forms. These products can be eaten, drunk, smoked, and vaped. Marijuana contains varying levels of delta-9-tetrahydrocannabinol (THC), the component responsible for euphoria and intoxication, and cannabidiol (CBD). While CBD is not intoxicating and does not lead to addiction, its long-term effects are largely unknown, and most CBD products are untested and of uncertain purity."*

When we read, "its long term effects are largely unknown," this

79 *Multiple Trump Administration Officials Speak Out Against Cannabis* Written by Johnny Green INTERNATIONAL CBC August 29, 2019

statement is true, but only in a certain context. Because research has been obstructed by the federal government, few "gold-standard clinical trials" have been conducted. So, in this sense it's effects are not fully known. However, millions of people have used this drug for *thousands of years*. So, considering this fact, this is a false statement.

Yet, we know the negative, and physical effects of alcohol. Despite this, the government allows it's sale. But no similar harms have been observed with cannabis.

Higher Potency Strains

The Surgeon General warns about higher potency cannabis. We read:

"Marijuana has changed over time. The marijuana available today is much stronger than previous versions. The THC concentration in commonly cultivated marijuana plants has increased three-fold between 1995 and 2014 (4% and 12% respectively). Marijuana available in dispensaries in some states has average concentrations of THC between 17.7% and 23.2%. Concentrated products, commonly known as dabs or waxes, are far more widely available to recreational users today and may contain between 23.7% and 75.9% THC."

The Surgeon General makes another misstatement, although likely unintentional. While it is true that access to higher potency cannabis strains has increased, these are *percentages related to availability*. Through selective breeding, strains with higher percentages of THC are now easier to obtain. You could find these strains in the 1960's or '70's, but it was rare.

What is not true, is that cannabis strains exist now that never existed before. The statement "marijuana has changed over time," attempts to assert this. It would be more accurate to write: *"stronger marijuana strains are more available now."*

While a case could be made that concentrates such as wax, shatter, or "live resin," were not available in previous years (although the process was known,) there is no evidence using a higher percentage of THC does any additional harm. Instead, the consumer of these higher strains adjusts to the "high." This has been observed in a clinical setting:

"Smoking high-potency marijuana concentrates boosts blood levels of THC more than twice as much as smoking conventional weed, but it doesn't necessarily get you higher, according to a new study of regular users published today by CU Boulder researchers. "Surprisingly, we found that potency did not track with intoxication levels," said lead author Cinnamon Bidwell, an assistant professor in the Institute of Cognitive Science. "While we saw striking differences in blood levels between the two groups, they were similarly impaired." The paper, published today in JAMA Psychiatry, is the first to assess the acute impact of cannabis among real-world users of legal market products. It, and more studies to come from the CUChange lab, could inform everything from roadside sobriety tests to decisions about personal recreational or medicinal use."[80]

Here are some of the details of this study:

"Findings In this cohort study of 121 cannabis flower users and concentrate users randomly assigned to higher- vs lower-THC products within user groups, use of legal market cannabis concentrates (ranging from 70%-90% tetrahydrocannabinol [THC]) produced significantly higher THC blood plasma levels compared with use of legal market cannabis flower (ranging from 16%-24% THC). Despite differences in THC exposure, flower and concentrate users showed similar neurobehavioral patterns after acute cannabis use and the domains of verbal memory and proprioception-focused postural stability for both groups were associated with THC." [81]

These researchers found *no difference* in "neurobehavioral impairments" between people who routinely used to low potency cannabis, or higher potency strains, and concentrates. This contrasts with the alarmist warnings of the Surgeon General. Compared to alcohol, THC is the weaker drug. The *more* you drink alcohol, the *more* you become impaired, sometimes fatally. Cannabis users develop a tolerance much quicker. The body adjusts to these amounts, so more THC does not necessarily equate to greater impairment. It can, but not with people who have developed tolerance to these stronger products.

Furthermore, people have consumed products with similar THC content for *thousands of years*. Hashish tests an average of 40 percent. Despite this high percentage, no difference in psychological functions has ever been observed.

Physical Dependence

"The risks of physical dependence, addiction, and other negative consequences increase with exposure to high concentrations of THC and the younger the age of initiation."

80 *Marijuana concentrates sharply spike THC levels but don't necessarily get users higher.* By Lisa Marshall. CU BOULDER TODAY. June 10, 2020
81 *Association of Naturalistic Administration of Cannabis Flower and Concentrates With Intoxication and Impairment.* JAMA PSYCHIATRY. June 10, 2020

The claim that addiction to cannabis occurs because stronger concentrates are being used has never been proven, as the claim that cannabis causes "physical dependence." This is also untrue, unless the word "dependence" is redefined. According to the National Institute of Drug Abuse (NIDA), this term means:

> "Physical Dependence: An adaptive physiological state that occurs with regular drug use and results in a withdrawal syndrome when drug use is stopped; often occurs with tolerance. Physical dependence can happen with chronic—even appropriate—use of many medications, and by itself does not constitute addiction.[82]"

According to the definition given by NIDA, Cannabis is not physically addicting, as opiates, or tranquilizers. This is confirmed by information released by the National Cancer Institute:

> "Although cannabinoids are considered by some to be addictive drugs, their addictive potential is considerably lower than that of other prescribed agents or substances of abuse.[2,4] The brain develops a tolerance to cannabinoids. Withdrawal symptoms such as irritability, insomnia with sleep electroencephalogram disturbance, restlessness, hot flashes, and, rarely, nausea and cramping have been observed. However, these symptoms appear to be mild compared with withdrawal symptoms associated with opiates or benzodiazepines, and the symptoms usually dissipate after a few days. "[83]

The claim of "physical addiction" is footnoted to a study titled: "***Examining the profile of high-potency cannabis and its association with severity of cannabis dependence***" from *Psychological Medicine*. It is a psychology journal. Nowhere in this study does it a claim cannabis is physically addicting. No physical tests were performed by these researchers; it is an analysis based on a self-survey. So, a "footnote trick" is being played on the reader. The reader thinks that the Surgeon General presents a footnote that proves cannabis causes physical addiction, but instead it purports psychological dependence. Of course, anyone can be psychologically addicted to any substance, even social media or cheesecake. Alcohol however, *can* cause physical addiction with extreme misuse. Addiction to alcohol begins psychological, but can become physical. Sudden withdraw can cause Delirium Tremens (DTs). This condition causes mania, hallucinations, and sometimes death.

The government has no problem with the legalization of alcohol. If

---

82 ***Classification and definition of misuse, abuse, and related events in clinical trials: ACTTION systematic review and recommendations*** HHS PUBLIC ACCESS. PUBMED. June 20, 2013
83 ***Cannabis and Cannabinoids (PDQ®)–Health Professional Version***.
NATIONAL CANCER INSTITUTE

"physical dependence" were a reason to keep cannabis illegal, prohibition of alcohol should return. Trump's donation has financed lies. Cannabis causes no one to become "physically dependent." It can have physical *symptoms* upon sudden withdraw, but so can caffeine.

Numerous prescription medications can cause *real* physical addiction, even when it is used as the Doctor prescribes. Here is a list of these government approved drugs:

1. All μ-opioids
2. Alcohol
3. Barbiturates such as phenobarbital, sodium thiopental and secobarbital
4. Benzodiazepines such as diazepam (Valium), lorazepam (Ativan), and alprazolam (Xanax)
5. Non-benzodiazepine hypnotics (z-drugs) such as zopiclone and zolpidem.
6. Gamma-hydroxybutyric acid (GHB) and 1,4-butanediol carisoprodol (Soma) and related carbamates (tybamate and meprobamate)
7. Baclofen (Lioresal)
8. Chloral hydrate
9. Glutethimide
10. Clomethiazole
11. Methaqualone (Quaalude)
12. Nicotine (tobacco)
13. Gabapentinoids such as gabapentin (Neurontin), pregabalin (Lyrica), and phenibut (Noofen)
14. Antipsychotic drugs such as clozapine, risperidone, olanzapine, haloperidol, thioridazine, etc.
15. Commonly prescribed antidepressants such as the selective serotonin reuptake inhibitors (SSRIs) and serotonin-norepinephrine reuptake inhibitors (SNRIs)
16. Blood pressure medications, including beta blockers such as propanolol and alpha-adrenergic agonists such as clonidine
17. Androgenic-anabolic steroids
18. Glucocorticoids

The law should be consistent. People lose respect for the law, if it is hypocritical. Unlike the false claim posted by the Surgeon General's office, these drugs are physically addicting. The Surgeon General uses the term "physical dependence" to scare the reader into supporting cannabis prohibition—but has no problem with any of these physically addicting prescription drugs.

<h2 align="center">"Psychosis"</h2>

The Surgeon General claims cannabis causes "psychosis." We read:

"Higher doses of THC are more likely to produce anxiety, agitation, paranoia, and psychosis."

This statement must be analyzed in the proper context. If a subject in these studies has *no* experience with cannabis, it can temporarily cause "anxiety, agitation, and paranoia." *For less than an hour.* Furthermore, the claim that "higher doses" cause these effects (more than lower dose cannabis) is a guess; it has never been proven. People with no tolerance can suffer these negative side effects regardless of cannabis strength.

The next claim—that cannabis causes *psychosis*—is only true if this term is redefined. In a 2016, the DEA honestly distinguishes between the various definitions of "psychosis," and *denies* cannabis causes this condition:

"This analysis evaluates only the evidence for a direct link between prior marijuana use and the subsequent development of psychosis. Thus, this discussion does not consider issues such as whether marijuana's transient effects are similar to psychotic symptoms in healthy individuals or exacerbate psychotic symptoms in individuals already diagnosed with schizophrenia. Extensive research has been conducted to investigate whether exposure to marijuana is associated with the development of schizophrenia or other psychoses. Although many studies are small and inferential, other studies in the literature use hundreds to thousands of subjects. At present, the available data do not suggest a causative link between marijuana use and the development of psychosis (Minozzi et al., 2010). Numerous large, longitudinal studies show that subjects who used marijuana do not have a greater incidence of psychotic diagnoses compared to those who do not use marijuana ..."[84]

The DEA distinguishes between "transient effects similar to psychotic symptoms" and *psychosis itself*. This is honest, unlike the Surgeon General's warning financed by President Trump. Some researchers who set out to discover the dangers of cannabis, hyper-define "psychosis." Instead of a permanent mental condition, they use this term to describe any temporary state of paranoia experienced by people who have no experience with the drug. The DEA refutes <u>the Surgeon General.</u>

84 ***Denial of Petition To Initiate Proceedings To Reschedule Marijuana***
DEPARTMENT OF JUSTICE Drug Enforcement Administration 21 CFR Chapter II [Docket No. DEA–426] Federal Register/Vol. 81, No. 156 / Friday, August 12, 2016

Overdose

Next, the Surgeon General claims cannabis can cause overdose:

"Edible marijuana takes time to absorb and to produce its effects, increasing the risk of unintentional overdose, as well as accidental ingestion by children and adolescents."

When many people read the word "overdose," they believe it means "death." Instead, it means, "taking more than intended." You can "overdose" on cheesecake, but it won't kill you. You will only get a stomach ache. Cannabis will not kill you either. It has caused zero overdose deaths. Paranoia, and falling asleep, are usually the only symptoms of a cannabis overdose. In rare instances with young children, breathing has been slightly suppressed after extreme amounts were consumed. But unlike opiates, breathing has never stopped. No children have died.

Yet, many of these over the counter drugs can cause "overdose deaths":

Midol
Tylenol
Advil
Epsom salts
Cough Syrup[85]

Children die from accidental ingestion of these common drugs all of the time. And of course, all prescription drugs that are potentially physically addicting can cause overdose deaths. So, the Surgeon General is using an excuse to continue cannabis prohibition. Alcohol is a legal intoxicant, and hundreds of kids die from alcohol poisoning every year.

Cannabinoid Hyperemesis Syndrome

Next, the Surgeon General warns about "Cannabinoid Hyperemesis Syndrome":

"In addition, chronic users of marijuana with a high THC content are at risk for developing a condition known as cannabinoid hyperemesis syndrome, which is marked by severe cycles of nausea and vomiting."

The Surgeon General's claim that "chronic users of marijuana with a high THC content" are at risk for developing cannabinoid hyperemesis syndrome has been debunked. A hair analysis of people who suffered from this condition

85 *5 common, over-the-counter medicines that could kill you if you take too much*
By Emily Cummings. NEWS 5 CLEVELAND. March 15, 2017_

indicate that they did *not* have extremely high levels of THC in their system:

> "Adults with an emergency department visit diagnosed as cannabis hyperemesis syndrome, near-daily use of cannabis for ≥6 months, and ≥2 episodes of severe vomiting in the previous year were age- and sex-matched to two control groups: RU controls (recreational users without vomiting), and ED controls (patients in the emergency department for an unrelated condition). Δ9-Tetrahydrocannabinol (THC), cannabinol (CBN), cannabidiol, and 11-nor-9-carboxy-THC concentrations in scalp hair were compared for subjects with positive urine THC. Results: We obtained satisfactory hair samples from 46 subjects with positive urine THC: 16 cases (age 26.8 ± 9.2 years; 69% male), 16 RU controls and 14 ED controls. Hair cannabinoid concentrations were similar between all three groups (e.g. cases THC 220 [median; IQR 100,730] pg/mg hair, RU controls 150 [71,320] and ED controls 270 [120,560]). Only the THC:CBN ratio was different between groups, with a 2.6-fold (95%CI 1.3,5.7) lower age- and sex-adjusted ratio in cases than RU controls. Hair cannabidiol concentrations were often unquantifiably low in all subjects." [86]

The footnote provided by the Surgeon General cites one of the first studies performed on this subject. These researchers go out of their way to distinguish between cannabinoid hyperemesis syndrome (CHS), and another disease—cyclic vomiting syndrome (CVS). Instead, the two illnesses could be closely related. They write:

> "In clinical practice CHS is most often confused with cyclic vomiting syndrome (CVS). In fact patients with CHS are often mislabeled as having CVS and vice versa. Confusion exists in the medical literature secondary to a failure to recognize chronic marijuana use as a source of vomiting. For example, in two recently published series of adult patients with CVS, approximately one third of patients reported daily marijuana use [65,66]. Based on the categorization of functional disorders developed by Rome III, chronic marijuana use (CHS) is recognized as a mechanism for nausea and vomiting distinct from CVS [67]. Although both conditions share an astonishing similarity, there are several significant differences. For example, CVS patients usually have important psychological comorbidities including depression and anxiety [64,65]. In addition, CVS patients have a high prevalence of migraine headaches or a family history of migraines. Furthermore, gastric emptying rates in patients

<hr>

86 *Hair cannabinoid concentrations in emergency patients with cannabis hyperemesis syndrome.* PUBMED. July 29, 2019

with CVS are often accelerated rather than delayed [46,65]. Table 2 summarizes some of the epidemiological and clinical characteristics that may help distinguish CVS and CHS.[87]"

Upon closer examination, all of these purported differences can be easily explained, and two of them are errors. First, they claim people with cyclic vomiting syndrome (CVS) do not take hot showers to relieve their symptoms. This is untrue. From *Rare Diseases*, we read:

> "The nausea and vomiting that characterize these episodes are often quite severe. Nausea can be persistent and intense. Unlike most other gastrointestinal disorders, the vomiting in CVS does not typically relieve the nausea. Affected children may experience bouts of rapid-fire, projectile vomiting as frequently as four or more times per hour with a peak pace of every 5-15 minutes. After the contents of the stomach are emptied, individuals may continue to dry heave. Symptoms can be so severe that affected individuals are unable to walk or talk and in some cases may appear unconscious or comatose. Episodes may cause affected individuals to withdraw from social interaction. The behavior of drinking water to dilute the bile and induce vomiting and hence reduce nausea is common, and should not be confused with a psychogenic cause. More commonly described in adults but also occurring in children, many take continuous prolonged hot shower or baths to alleviate the nausea." (Cyclic Vomiting Syndrome. RARE DISEASES.org[88])

Some people who suffer from CVS do take hot showers to relieve their symptoms. However, since this fact has escaped these researchers, it could be that some suffer from it, while others do not. Likewise, not everyone who suffers from cannabinoid hyperemesis syndrome (CHS) might not feel the need to relieve their symptoms in this manner. People are genetically different.

Another cited "difference" might also be subjective. We read:

> "...other differences...CVS patients have a high prevalence of migraine headaches or a family history of migraines"

Their claim that CHS patients do not suffer from migraines is also incorrect. According to a case report a man with CHS *did* suffer from a headache:

> "The patient was admitted to the hospital and immediately treated with intravenous fluids, including normal saline (2 L bolus

87 *Cannabinoid Hyperemesis Syndrome* CURRENT DRUG ABUSE REVIEWS. PUBMED. December 4, 2011

88 *Cyclic Vomiting Syndrome*. RARE DISEASES.ORG

and then 200 mL/hr) and famotidine (20 mg). Within the next 2 hours, the patient experienced minimal relief as we administered ondansetron hydrochloride for nausea and vomiting (4 mg as needed), morphine for pain (4 mg as needed), droperidol (5 mg), diphenhydramine hydrochloride (50 mg), promethazine hydrochloride (12.5 mg as needed), chlorpromazine hydrochloride for resolution of intractable hiccups (25 mg as needed), and acetaminophen for headache (650 mg as needed). Except for the acetaminophen, all drugs were administered intravenously. The patient vomited several times overnight and nausea was still present the next morning. However, the patient reported that his headache had resolved and abdominal pain was improving. In addition, the patient's dehydration, relative polycythemia, and leukocytosis had improved, and his hiccups had resolved. The patient took multiple hot showers on this day."[89]

This man had a migraine, despite the assertion of these researchers. But everyone might not suffer from this symptom, since cannabis treats migraines:

"We found that self-reported headache and migraine severity were reduced by nearly 50% from before to after cannabis use," said study author Carrie Cuttler. She is an assistant professor in the department of psychology at Washington State University in Pullman, Wash."[90]

So, this "difference" could also vary from person to person. Despite slightly dissimilar symptoms, people are genetically different. There could be a similar cause behind both illnesses.

Another stated "difference" is depression. People with CVS: "... usually have important psychological comorbidities including depression and anxiety" (but not cannabis users.) This "difference" can be explained by the antidepressant properties of cannabis:

"According to a research study published by the University Of New Mexico and Releaf App in the Yale The findings suggest that, at least in the short term, the vast majority of patients that use cannabis experience antidepressant effects, although the magnitude of the effect and extent of side effect experiences vary with chemotypic properties of the plant."[91]

89 *Cannabinoid Hyperemesis Syndrome as the Underlying Cause of Intractable Nausea and Vomiting*. The Journal of the American Osteopathic Association. March, 2011

90 *Cannabis Reduces Headache, Migraine Severity* by Nearly Half, Study Shows AJMC November 26, 2019_

91 *The Effectiveness of Cannabis Flower for Immediate Relief from Symptoms of Depression* PUBMED June, 2020

Another cited "difference" is with gastric emptying rates:

"...gastric emptying rates in patients with CVS are often accelerated rather than delayed..."

Once again, the medicinal properties of cannabis could explain this "difference." Cannabis can treat gastric diseases. From *Gastroenterology & Hepatology*, we read:

"The marijuana plant Cannabis sativa and its derivatives, cannabinoids, have grown increasingly popular as a potential therapy for inflammatory bowel disease (IBD). Studies have shown that modulation of the endocannabinoid system, which regulates various functions in the body and has been shown to play a key role in the pathogenesis of IBD, has a therapeutic effect in mouse colitis..."[92]

We also read from *Medical News Today*:

"Treatment with cannabis can relieve symptoms and improve quality of life in individuals with Crohn's disease even though it has no impact on gut inflammation, according to new research presented at a conference recently."[93]

Cannabis can treat bowel discomfort. This could explain why this symptom is not as pronounced in both groups. The only remaining "difference" cited are "triggering factors." In CVS patients, stress can trigger these symptoms. It does not *appear* to happen in people with CHS. However, cannabis could be a trigger itself. When these people quit using it, their symptoms go away[94].

---

92 ***Therapeutic Use of Cannabis in Inflammatory Bowel Disease*** GASTROENTEROLOGY & HEPATOLOGY PUBMED November 12, 2016

93 ***Cannabis relieves symptoms in Crohn's disease***. Medical News Today October 22, 2018

94 "The cannabinoid hyperemesis syndrome (CHS) and the cyclic vomiting syndrome in adults (CVS) are both characterized by recurrent episodes of heavy nausea, vomiting and frequently abdominal pain. Both syndromes are barely known among physicians. Literature is inconsistent concerning clinical features which enable differentiation between CVS and CHS. We performed a literature review using the LIVIVO search portal for life sciences to develop a pragmatic approach towards these two syndromes. Our findings indicate that complete and persistent resolution of all symptoms of the disease following cannabis cessation is the only reliable criterion applicable to distinguish CHS from CVS. Psychiatric comorbidities (e.g. panic attacks, depression), history of migraine attacks and rapid gastric emptying may serve as supportive criteria for the diagnosis of CVS. Compulsive bathing behaviour, a clinical observation previously attributed only to CHS patients is equally present in CVS patients. " (***Cannabinoid hyperemesis and the cyclic vomiting syndrome in adults: recognition, diagnosis, acute and long-term treatment.*** GERMAN MEDICAL SCIENCE. PUBMED. March 21, 2017

A Recent Phenomenon

The first case of cannabis hyperemesis syndrome was reported in 2004[95], a few years after the legalization of medical cannabis. This timing does not appear coincidental. Certain chemicals, fertilizers, insecticides, or anti fungals used in mass production *could* explain the sudden emergence of this disease due to allergies, or being more susceptible to these agents.

The hair analysis however, tells a different story. In these results, we likely discover the cause of this disease. There was *one* difference between these two groups. In a previous study, we read:

"Only the THC:CBN ratio was different between groups" [96]

CBN (Cannabinol) is not native to the cannabis plant, but is created when the cannabis plant gets old, and THC, and THCA degrades. These cannabinoids change into CBN inside of the plant, or CBN can be made by heat in an extraction process. In the latter case, the ratio of THC/CBN is usually about 1:1. So, the public consumption of *CBN* has suddenly changed. Prior to consistent, higher potency cannabis *sold in volume*, less plants were grown, containing less THC, which means less CBN was consumed.

Commercialized cannabis can suffer from over-supply, which usually means more cannabis stays on the shelf, and degrades—turning into "high potency CBN weed." This substance binds to at least two receptors in the human body responsible for the regulation of heat, touch, stomach, and every symptom of both CVS, and CHS.

The "TRPV Channels"

Scientists theorize that THC down-regulation of the TRPV1 gene causes CHS[97]. This hypothesis might stem from recent sales of high potency THC, or is simply an effort to make THC the "bad guy." But remember, *hair analysis* refutes this theory. TRPV1 is not the only gene that could, in theory, cause this illness. Other TRPV genes could be implicated. From *Current Pharmaceutical Biotechnology*, we read:

> "Several of the 28 mammalian transient receptor potential (TRP) channel subunits are expressed throughout the alimentary canal where they play important roles in taste, chemo- and mechanosensation, thermoregulation, pain and hyperalgesia,

95 ***Cannabinoid hyperemesis with the unusual symptom of compulsive bathing*** NEDERLANDS TIJDSCHRIFT VOOR GENEESKUNDE. PUBMED June, 2005

96 ***Hair cannabinoid concentrations in emergency patients with cannabis hyperemesis syndrome.*** CANADIAN JOURNAL OF EMERGENCY MEDICAL CARE. PUBMED. July 29, 2019

97 ***Successful Treatment of Cannabinoid Hyperemesis Syndrome with Topical Capsaicin*** ACG CASE REPORTS. PUBMED January 3, 2018

mucosal function and homeostasis, control of motility by neurons, interstitial cells of Cajal and muscle cells, and vascular function. While the implications of some TRP channels, notably TRPA1, TRPC4, TRPM5, TRPM6, TRPM7, TRPV1, TRPV4, and TRPV6, have been investigated in much detail, the understanding of other TRP channels in their relevance to digestive function lags behind. The polymodal chemo- and mechanosensory function of TRPA1, TRPM5, TRPV1 and TRPV4 is particularly relevant to the alimentary canal whose digestive and absorptive function depends on the surveillance and integration of many chemical and physical stimuli."[98]

Different cannabinoids bind to the TRPV channels in different ways. But there are four that likely play a role in this illness: TRPV1, TRPA1, TRPM5, and TRPV4. Because THC down regulates, and desensitizes the TRPV1 receptor, this is being investigated as a cause of hyperemesis. We read:

"There is a high density of TRPV1 receptors in the area postrema known as the "trigger zone" for emesis [22]. Endocannabinoids (anandamide) along with exogenous cannabinoids (cannabidiol [CBD], cannabidivarin) are TRPV1 agonists [23, 24]. To complicate the picture, TRPV1 agonism appears to be proemetic when ligand concentration is low, but antiemetic when ligand concentration is high [23, 24]. Extreme stimulation can desensitize TRPV1 and be proemetic [25]. TRPV1 desensitization may occur because signaling by substance P and CGRP has been disrupted, resulting in a lower density of substance P receptors in the brain regions associated with vomiting [25, 26]. Opening the TRPV1 channels may impair substance P signaling in the vomiting center of the brain by overstimulating TRPV1, which then results in antiemetic effects. Thus, desensitized TRPV1 receptors may promote emesis while opening TRPV1 channels may be antiemetic"[99]

Desensitizing this receptor causes vomiting, but "opening" it does the opposite. This is *only* one receptor *out of four* that can effect the human body in this manner. Two others are desensitized by *CBN*. From *Psysiologica*, we read:

"CBD, CBG, CBGV and THCV stimulated and desensitized human TRPV1. CBC, CBD and CBN were potent rat TRPA1 agonists and desensitizers, but THCV-BDS was the most potent compound at this target. CBG-BDS and THCV-BDS were the most potent rat TRPM8 antagonists. All non-acid cannabinoids, except CBC and

98 *TRP channels in the digestive system*.
CURRENT PHARMACEUTICAL BIOTECHNOLOGY. PUBMED January 1, 2011
99 *Cannabinoid Hyperemesis*. KARGER. January 2019

CBN, potently activated and desensitized rat TRPV2." (PUBMED[100])

We also read from *Frontiers in Mononuclear Neuroscience*:

"Concerning plant-derived cannabinoids, De Petrocellis et al. (2012a) discovered that specific compounds are also able to evoke intracellular Ca2+ response in cells expressing TRPV4. As depicted in Table Table4,4, phytogenic analogs of CBD and Δ9-THC bearing a propyl side chain, CBDV and THCV, showed the highest efficacy and potency among the phytocannabinoids tested. These results may prompt consideration of the structural importance of cannabinoid lipophilic side chains and their interactions at TRPV4. On the other hand, phytocannabinoids such as CBG, CBGA, CBGV, and CBN (Figure (Figure5)5) were more readily able to desensitize this channel (after activation by 4-α-phorbol-12,13-didecanoate, 4α-PDD), even though these phytocannabinoids exhibited low efficacy and/or potency as activators of this channel." [101]

TRPA1 is responsible for feeling cold, and pain. TRPV4 causes migraine headaches. CBN binds to, and desensitizes both of these two channels, while THC does this to TRPV1. If after hair tests, and these facts are taken into consideration, this illness is likely caused by CBN, combined with genetic mutations. Since age turns cannabis into high CBD/low THC flower, all *three* of these channels become desensitized at the same time, but *TRPV1 to a lesser extent*.

There appears to be an interaction, and/or overlap between cannabinoid, and TRP receptors. We read:

"To date, six TRP channels from the three subfamilies mentioned above have been reported to mediate cannabinoid activity: TRPV1, TRPV2, TRPV3, TRPV4, TRPA1, and TRPM8. The increasing data regarding cannabinoid interactions with these receptors has prompted some researchers to consider these TRP channels to be "ionotropic cannabinoid receptors." Although CB1 and CB2 are considered to be the canonical cannabinoid receptors, there is significant overlap between cannabinoids and ligands of TRP receptors."[102]

Other factors appear to be involved in this process. CBN, and THC bind to three of these receptors, but only inhibiting two of these *abolishes* calcium

100 ***Cannabinoid actions at TRPV channels: Effects on TRPV3 and TRPV4 and their potential relevance to gastrointestinal inflammation*** ACTA PSYSIOLOGICA. RESEARCH GATE. July 2011.
101 ***Cannabinoid Ligands Targeting TRP Channels*** FRONTIERS IN MOLECULAR NEUROSCIENCE. PUBMED. January 15, 2019
102 ***idib***

channel responses:

> "...we discovered that across all neurons were Ca2+ responses were diminished (averaged across all neurons) with knockout/ inhibition of either TRPA1 or TRPV1 and largely abolished with dual knockout/inhibition of both channels."[103]

Together CBN, and THC inhibits, or "knocks out" *both* of these channels. However, genetics cause people to become susceptible; the majority of people do not get sick from older cannabis, high in CBN.

Mutations in the Mitochondrial DNA could also contribute to these symptoms, and inhibition of the TRPV channels is related to mitochondria dysfunction. A complex series of events are the likely cause of CHS, and CVS. As we read, stress is a trigger of CHS. Stress also contributes to mitochondrial dysfunction. From *Rare Diseases*, we read:

> "Researchers have also learned that blood and urine testing reveals signs of abnormal energy metabolism. Changes (mutations) in genetic material found in the mitochondrial DNA (mtDNA) may play a role in the development of CVS but reducing the capacity to produce sufficient energy during times of stress such as fever, illness, hot weather (sweating), excitement and aerobic exercise. Because mitochondria (cell's power plant) in particular power muscle and nerve tissue, defective mitochondrial energy production may lead to a energy shortage during stress that affects nerve function, especially the autonomic nerves that control the gut."[104]

Stress can act as a "trigger," causing CVS. Researchers found this affects the mitochondria. This "dysfunction" can also be caused by almost *every* drug— *including THC*. From the *Journal of Biomedicine, and Biotechnology,* we read:

> "...THC significantly enhanced H2O2 production by cerebral mitochondria (+171%; P < 0.05) and mitochondrial free radical leak was increased from 0.01±0.01 to 0.10±0.01% (P < 0.001). Thus, THC increases oxidative stress and induces cerebral mitochondrial dysfunction."[105]

THC contributes to mitochondrial dysfunction. But so does alcohol,

103 *Integrative Signaling of Mitochondria, TRPA1 and TRPV1 in Vagal Neurons* UNIVERSITY OF SOUTH FLORIDA. 2018

104 *Cyclic Vomiting Syndrome.* RARE DISEASES.org

105 *Tetrahydrocannbinol Induces Brain Mitochondrial Respiratory Chain Dysfunction and Increases Oxidative Stress: A Potential Mechanism Involved in Cannabis-Related Stroke.* JOURNAL OF BIOMEDICINE AND BIOTECHNOLOGY. PUBMED January 14, 2015

opiates, and many over the counter drugs. People with a specific genetic issue are susceptible to certain agents, or stimuli, causing a cascade of physical events.

Deaths from Cannabinoid Hyperemesis Syndrome

CVS has caused a few deaths. It is curious the Surgeon General did not post anything about these deaths—unless there is a plan to create commercials later. Perhaps we will see grieving parents talking about their dead kids, prior to an industry-wide shutdown. If they use this tactic, they are being disingenuous, because this rarely occurs. Yet, if dehydration from vomiting is cause for keeping a drug off of the market, what about alcohol? Statistically, there are higher incidences of alcohol induced hyperemesis. And, this vomiting can be severe. We read:

> "Untreated severe dehydration from vomiting can cause seizures, permanent brain damage, or death. Even if the victim lives, an alcohol overdose can lead to irreversible brain damage. Rapid binge drinking (which often happens on a bet or a dare) is especially dangerous because the victim can ingest a fatal dose before becoming unconscious."[106]

Dehydration from alcohol kills more people than dehydration from CHS. The few fatalities from dehydration occurred only in a subset of people who have a specific genetic condition. *Anyone* can be affected by alcohol this way, when drinking too much.

CBD Oil and the Mitochondria

CBD acts on different receptors than THC, and also independent of these receptors. While THC, and CBN cause dysfunction the mitochondria, CBD appears to have the opposite effect. From *Science Direct*, we read.

> "Cannabidiol (CBD) is a nonpsychoactive cannabinoid derived from Cannabis sativa and a weak CB1 and CB2 cannabinoid receptor antagonist, with very low toxicity for humans. It has recently been demonstrated in vivo and in vitro that CBD has a variety of therapeutic properties, exerting antidepressant, anxiolytic, anti-inflammatory, immunomodulatory, and neuroprotective effects [4]. Increasing evidence indicates that CBD is a molecule with potentially neuroprotective properties that can be used to treat neurodegenerative disorders. CBD had been shown to reverse the reduction in neuronal viability and the increased excitoxicity, inflammation, and oxidative stress in newborn piglets with hypoxic–ischemic brain damage by targeting the

receptors of 5HT1A and CB2[5]; and to protect PC12 and SH-SYS5 cells from tert-butyl-hydroperoxide-induced oxidative stress, independently of the CB1 and CB2 receptors [6]. CBD also displays better protective activity against glutamate neurotoxicity than either ascorbate or alpha-tocopherol, which suggests that it is a potentially effective antioxidant [7]. ... Our results provide novel insight into the neuroprotective properties of CBD, which involves the regulation of the mitochondrial bioenergetics and the glucose metabolism of hippocampal neurons during OGD/R injury."[107]

In this study on neurodegeneration, we discover that CBD is a powerful cannabinoid, with anti-oxidant effects. It can reduce inflammation, and *regulate* the mitochondria. Whether this effect is strong enough to counteract the effects CHS, is unknown.

Mitochondrial Dysfunction, Cannabis and Strokes

Several news reports have linked cannabis use to a few strokes in young people. This is a case study of one such event:

"Abstract Drug misuse represents a risk factor for cerebrovascular disease, especially among young people. Despite the fact that cannabis is the most widely used illicit drug, there are only a few reports associating its use with cerebrovascular disease. We describe a patient who suffered three ischaemic strokes immediately after cannabis consumption. Other stroke aetiologies were ruled out, and neuroimaging revealed infarcts in different arterial areas as well as evidence of non-atherosclerotic arterial disease, which suggests an underlying vasculopathy of uncertain (toxic or inflammatory) origin. Cannabis use may be associated with ischaemic stroke in young patients, but its mechanism is unclear."[108]

Regarding the connection between cannabis, and strokes, these researchers admit the "mechanism is unclear," and admit that there are only a *few reports*. This is similar to people with mitochondrial dysfunction. A few of these people have strokes *without* cannabis use. From the periodical *Stroke*, we read:

---

107 *Cannabidiol attenuates OGD/R-induced damage by enhancing mitochondrial bioenergetics and modulating glucose metabolism via pentose-phosphate pathway in hippocampal neurons.* SCIENCE DIRECT. April, 2017.

108 *Recurrent stroke associated with cannabis use* JOURNAL OF NEUROLOGY, NEUROSURGERY, AND PSYCHIATRY. PUBMED February 16, 2005

"It is well known that some mitochondrial disorders are responsible for ischemic cerebral infarction in young patients. Our purpose was to determine, in this prospective ongoing study, whether ischemic stroke is the only manifestation of a mitochondrial disorder in young patients.

Methods—Patients aged ≤50 years, admitted to the Stroke Unit from January 1999 to May 2000 with a diagnosis of ischemic stroke of unknown origin, were included in the study. All of them had full biochemical and hematologic tests, neuroimaging studies, transesophageal echocardiography, and extracranial and transcranial Doppler sonography. Patent foramen ovale was ruled out. Lactic acid concentrations were measured after anaerobic exercise of the forearm, and a morphological, biochemical, and molecular study after biceps muscle biopsy was performed. Results— Of the 18 patients so far included, 3 (17%) presented lactic acid hyperproduction after physical exercise, and 6 (33%) showed deficit of the mitochondrial respiratory chain complexes. The molecular analyses have confirmed mitochondrial mutations at base pairs 3243 (characteristic of mitochondrial encephalomyopathy, lactic acidosis, and strokelike episodes [MELAS]), 4216, and 15 928. Conclusions—These results suggest that ischemic stroke may be the only manifestation or the initial manifestation of a mitochondrial disorder."[109]

It is possible the same rare condition that can cause strokes also contributes to CHS and CVS. As stress can trigger a stroke with Mitochondrial dysfunction, so could cannabis. Someone who does not have this genetic disease however, will not suffer a stroke after either event.

These connections are there for everyone to see, but because researchers are bias against cannabis, they have missed this evidence—*as the Surgeon General*.

Cannabis Hyperemesis Syndrome Successfully Treated

Scientists in India have found a treatment for cannabinoid hyperemesis syndrome. This treatment itself is evidence mitochondrial dysfunction plays a role in this disease. Success was achieved after the patient was treated with the prescription drug haloperidol. From *Case Reports in Psychiatry*, we read:

"Chronic use of cannabis can result in a syndrome of hyperemesis characterized by cyclical vomiting without any other identifiable causes. Cannabinoid hyperemesis syndrome (CHS) is seldom responsive to traditional antiemetic therapies. Despite frequent nausea and vomiting, patients may be reluctant to discontinue

---

109 *Mitochondrial Disease and Stroke*. STROKE. AHA JOURNALS. November 2001

use of cannabis. We report a case of severe, refractory CHS with complete resolution of nausea and vomiting after treatment with haloperidol in the outpatient setting. After review of the literature, we believe this is the first reported successful outpatient treatment of CHS and suggests a potential treatment for refractory patients."[110]

This drug made the symptoms of cannabis hyperemesis syndrome disappear. This was discovered in 2016. So, why didn't physicians use this drug in several subsequent cases that have caused fatalities? Were they so overwhelmed with information they were not able to do a simple search of the database?

Guess what Haloperidol inhibits? The Mitochondria. From the International Journal of Neuropharmacology, we read:

"We have examined the effects of a variety of classical and atypical neuroleptic drugs on mitochondrial NADH ubiquinone oxido-reductase (complex I) activity. Sagittal slices of mouse brain incubated in vitro with haloperidol (10 nM) showed time- and concentration-dependent inhibition of complex I. Similar concentrations of the pyridinium metabolite of haloperidol (HPP+) failed to inhibit complex I activity in this model; indeed, comparable inhibition was obtained only at a 10000-fold higher concentration of HPP+ (100 microM). Treatment of brain slices with haloperidol resulted in a loss of glutathione (GSH), while pretreatment of slices with GSH and alpha-lipoic acid abolished haloperidol-induced loss of complex I activity. Incubation of mitochondria from haloperidol treated brain slices with the thiol reductant, dithiothreitol, completely regenerated complex I activity demonstrating thiol oxidation as a feasible mechanism of inhibition. In a comparison of different neuroleptic drugs, haloperidol was the most potent inhibitor of complex I, followed by chlorpromazine, fluphenazine and risperidone while the atypical neuroleptic, clozapine (100 microM) did not inhibit complex I activity in mouse brain slices. The present studies support the view that classical neuroleptics such as haloperidol inhibit mitochondrial complex I through oxidative modification of the enzyme complex."[111]

A drug that inhibits the mitochondria successfully treated cannabis hyperemesis syndrome, which is evidence this disease is related to a dysfunction of the mitochondria.

---

110 *Successful Treatment of Suspected Cannabinoid Hyperemesis Syndrome Using Haloperidol in the Outpatient Setting* CASE REPORTS IN PSYCHIATRY. PUBMED. August 11, 2016
111 *Inhibition of mitochondrial complex I by haloperidol: the role of thiol oxidation.* INTERNATIONAL JOURNAL OF NEUROPHARMACOLOGY. PUBMED April 1999

These observations—about the role CBN in this disease—would be easy to test. Researchers could have Haloperidol on hand, in case of a reaction. People who suffered from CHS could be recruited in a study, and given intravenous THC. If this does not cause CHS, call them back another day, and give them CBN. If this triggers a reaction, the cause of this disease is proven.

Cannabis and Heart Attacks

Although not mentioned in the Surgeon General's warning, recent studies attempt to connect cannabis use with heart attacks. These studies are usually based only on interviews, and are fodder for the news media. For instance, we read from *Healthline* in 2017:

> "When it comes to heart health, is marijuana any safer for you than tobacco? A new study published today in the European Journal of Preventive Cardiology concluded that marijuana use is associated with a threefold risk of death from hypertension. "This is not surprising since marijuana is known to have a number of effects on the cardiovascular system. Marijuana stimulates the sympathetic nervous system, leading to increases in heart rate, blood pressure, and oxygen demand," said Barbara A. Yankey, study lead author, and PhD student in the School of Public Health at Georgia State University, in a press statement. Their results were based on a specially designed retrospective study. Researchers analyzed data from 1,213 participants who were considered marijuana users based on their responses to the 2005-2006 National Health and Nutrition Examination Survey (NHANES). This data was cross referenced with mortality data from 2011 from the National Center for Health Statistics." [112]

Many anti-cannabis activists quoted from this news story, and it is still referenced today. Many doubted it at the time, stating that it used bad methodology. This news story is still online, repeated in multiple outlets, which all reference the research. The problem? The journal that published the study has retracted it, due to skewed statistical data. From *Sage Publications*, we read:

> "At the request of the Journal Editor and SAGE Publishing, with the agreement of the authors, the following article has been retracted. Yankey B.A., Rothenberg R, S. Ramsey-White K and Okosun I S. Effect of marijuana use on cardiovascular and cerebrovascular mortality: A study using the National Heath and Nutrition Examination Survey linked mortality file. European Journal of Preventive Cardiology 2017; 24; 1833-1840 DOI: 10.1177/2047487317723212. A methodological error has led to

112 ***Study on Marijuana and Heart Health Stirs Debate.*** HEALTHLINE. August 16, 2017

immortality bias within the findings of this article; therefore, the survival intervals for participants used in this survey were unsound. Any patients who died prior to 2005 would not have been able to posthumously complete the survey regarding marijuana use. As such it is not possible to ascertain the marijuana use of patients who died prior to 2005. As a result, survival status prior to the completion of the survey should have been censored."[113]

This study used data complied by the "National Health and Nutrition Examination Survey." *NHANES* is conducted by the Centers for Disease Control (CDC). European researchers reanalyzed this data, and concluded the results were skewed, because questions were answered about marijuana on behalf of the dead.

Many of these studies assume cannabis increases blood pressure. This is true only with first use. After a tolerance to these effects, hypotension occurs[114]. So, any extrapolation of continued hypertension in these studies, and it's continued damage on the heart, and cardiovascular system, is incorrect.

Another study linking cannabis to heart attacks honestly admits to it's limitations. From *Circulation*, we read:

> "A key concern is whether cannabis triggers or potentiates major adverse cardiovascular events such as AMI and arrhythmias, as well as its impact on cardiovascular risk factors. Unfortunately, most of the available data are short term, observational, and retrospective in nature; lack exposure determination; exhibit recall bias; include minimal cannabis exposure with no dose or

---

113 *RETRACTED: Effect of marijuana use on cardiovascular and cerebrovascular mortality: A study using the National Health and Nutrition Examination Survey linked mortality file.* SAGE PUBLICATIONS

114 "Marijuana and delta9-tetrahydrocannabinol (THC) increase heart rate, slightly increase supine blood pressure, and on occasion produce marked orthostatic hypotension. Cardiovascular effects in animals are different, with bradycardia and hypotension the most typical response. Cardiac output increases, and peripheral vascular resistance and maximum exercise performance decrease. Tolerance to most of the initial cardiovascular effects appears rapidly. With repeated exposure, supine blood pressure decreases slightly, orthostatic hypotension disappears, blood volume increases, heart rate slows, and circulatory responses to exercise and Valsalva maneuver are diminished, consistent with centrally mediated, reduced sympathetic, and enhanced parasympathetic activity. Receptor-mediated and probably nonneuronal sites of action account for cannabinoid effects. The endocannabinoid system appears important in the modulation of many vascular functions. Marijuana's cardiovascular effects are not associated with serious health problems for most young, healthy users, although occasional myocardial infarction, stroke, and other adverse cardiovascular events are reported. Marijuana smoking by people with cardiovascular disease poses health risks because of the consequences of the resulting increased cardiac work, increased catecholamine levels, carboxyhemoglobin, and postural hypotension." https://pubmed.ncbi.nlm.nih.gov/12412837/

product standardization; and typically evaluate low-risk cohorts. In addition, many epidemiological studies may be confounded by factors associated with access to health care and other adverse health behaviors such as tobacco use. Finally, because the concentration of THC in cannabis has been increasing over the past several years, earlier studies may not be relevant to the present experience."[115]

According to this research, many factors confound the results. How studies are performed is also a factor. If someone goes to heart attack patients, they do not get a sample that represents the population. Studies that follow large groups of people, over long periods of time show *no correlation* between cannabis use and heart attacks. From the *American Journal of Public Health*, we read:

"Objectives: To investigate the effects of marijuana in the development of incident cardiovascular and cerebrovascular outcomes. Methods: Participants were 5113 adults aged 18 to 30 years at baseline (1985-1986) from the Coronary Artery Risk Development in Young Adults study, who were followed for more than 25 years. We estimated cumulative lifetime exposure to marijuana using repeated assessments collected at examinations every 2 to 5 years. The primary outcome was incident cardiovascular disease (CVD) through 2013. Results: A total of 84% (n = 4286) reported a history of marijuana use. During a median 26.9 years (131 990 person-years), we identified 215 CVD events, including 62 strokes or transient ischemic attacks, 104 cases of coronary heart disease, and 50 CVD deaths. Compared with no marijuana use, cumulative lifetime and recent marijuana use showed no association with incident CVD, stroke or transient ischemic attacks, coronary heart disease, or CVD mortality. Marijuana use was not associated with CVD when stratified by age, gender, race, or family history of CVD. Conclusions: Neither cumulative lifetime nor recent use of marijuana is associated with the incidence of CVD in middle age." (*Cumulative Lifetime Marijuana Use and Incident Cardiovascular Disease in Middle Age: The Coronary Artery Risk Development in Young Adults (CARDIA) Study*. PUBMED. April, 2017)[116]

This study looked at a sample more representative of the population, and found no link between cannabis use and heart attacks. Another study

---

115 *Medical Marijuana, Recreational Cannabis, and Cardiovascular Health*. CIRCULATION. AHA JOURNALS. September 8, 2020.

116 *Cumulative Lifetime Marijuana Use and Incident Cardiovascular Disease in Middle Age: The Coronary Artery Risk Development in Young Adults (CARDIA) Study*. AMERICAN JOURNAL OF PUBLIC HEALTH. PUBMED. April, 2017

concluded that the only negative health effect of Cannabis was bad teeth. From the *Journal of the American Medical Association Psychiatry*, we read:

> "We tested whether cannabis use from ages 18 to 38 years was associated with physical health at age 38, even after controlling for tobacco use, childhood health, and childhood socioeconomic status. We also tested whether cannabis use from ages 26 to 38 years was associated with within-individual health decline using the same measures of health at both ages. Exposures: We assessed frequency of cannabis use and cannabis dependence at ages 18, 21, 26, 32, and 38 years. Main outcomes and measures: We obtained laboratory measures of physical health (periodontal health, lung function, systemic inflammation, and metabolic health), as well as self-reported physical health, at ages 26 and 38 years. Results: The 1037 study participants were 51.6% male (n = 535). Of these, 484 had ever used tobacco daily and 675 had ever used cannabis. Cannabis use was associated with poorer periodontal health at age 38 years and within-individual decline in periodontal health from ages 26 to 38 years. For example, cannabis joint-years from ages 18 to 38 years was associated with poorer periodontal health at age 38 years, even after controlling for tobacco pack-years (β = 0.12; 95% CI, 0.05-0.18; P <.001). Additionally, cannabis joint-years from ages 26 to 38 years was associated with poorer periodontal health at age 38 years, even after accounting for periodontal health at age 26 years and tobacco pack-years (β = 0.10; 95% CI, 0.05-0.16; P <.001) However, cannabis use was unrelated to other physical health problems. Unlike cannabis use, tobacco use was associated with worse lung function, systemic inflammation, and metabolic health at age 38 years, as well as within-individual decline in health from ages 26 to 38 years. Conclusions and relevance: Cannabis use for up to 20 years is associated with periodontal disease but is not associated with other physical health problems in early midlife. Conflict of interest statement. The authors have no conflicts of interest to report. MHM had full access to all the data in the study and takes responsibility for the integrity of thedata and the accuracy of the data analysis."[117]

Studies that looked at larger, more accurate samples found no link between cannabis use, and strokes or heart attacks. However, this has occurred on rare occasions. From *Cardiology in the Young*, we read:

---

117 *Associations Between Cannabis Use and Physical Health Problems in Early Midlife: A Longitudinal Comparison of Persistent Cannabis vs Tobacco Users.* JOURNAL OF THE AMERICAN MEDICAL ASSOCIATION PSYCHIATRY. PUBMED. July, 2016

"Cannabis smoking is considered the most popular illicit drug used worldwide. We present the case of a 26-year-old male with ST elevation myocardial infarction and heart failure subsequent to cannabis smoking abuse. We searched the literature regarding acute myocardial infarction following cannabis smoking and the possible pathophysiologic mechanisms."[118]

So, if there have been cases of people who have had heart attacks with cannabis, should I be concerned? It depends if you suffer from *Mitochondrial dysfunction.* Even *without* cannabis use, this disease can cause heart attacks. From the *Annals of Translational Medicine,* we read:

"Mitochondrial dysfunction is associated with the development of numerous cardiac diseases such as atherosclerosis, ischemia-reperfusion (I/R) injury, hypertension, diabetes, cardiac hypertrophy and heart failure (HF), due to the uncontrolled production of reactive oxygen species (ROS). Therefore, early control of mitochondrial dysfunction is a crucial step in the therapy of cardiac diseases. A number of anti-oxidant molecules and medications have been used but the results are inconsistent among the studies. Eventually, the aim of future research is to design molecules which selectively target mitochondrial dysfunction and restore the capacity of cellular anti-oxidant enzymes."[119]

The same genetic condition that could be implicated in cannabinoid hyperemesis syndrome also can cause heart attacks. Therefore, if you have this disease, smoking cannabis puts you at risk. About a one in 100,000 chance of a heart attack or stroke. People who suffer from this condition should use cannabis with caution, or not at all.

Furthermore, people who suffer from high blood pressure could put themselves at risk, if they use cannabis everyday, and stop abruptly. From *Journal of Addiction Medicine,* we read:

"Abrupt cessation of heavy cannabis use may cause clinically significant increases in blood pressure in a subset of users. Blood pressure should be monitored among those attempting to reduce or quit frequent cannabis use, particularly those with preexisting hypertension. The time course of this effect is currently unknown

---

118 *ST elevation myocardial infarction following a cannabis smoking binge.* CARDIOLOGY IN THE YOUNG. PUBMED. July, 14, 2019

119 *Mitochondria and cardiovascular diseases—from pathophysiology to treatment.* ANNALS OF TRANSLATIONAL MEDICINE. PUBMED June 6, 2018

and requires further study. "[120]

If you suffer from high blood pressure, abruptly stopping any medication that controls it could cause a heart attack or stroke. Because cannabis causes hypotension with use, people with high blood pressure should never quit cannabis suddenly. In this regard, it could be dangerous. But only if someone suffers from hypertension.

But this should not be any reason to continue prohibition. The majority should not be criminalized, because the minority suffer from a medical condition. Alcohol can also cause heart attacks, with simple misuse. From *Johns Hopkins*, we read:

> "Heavy drinking, on the other hand, is linked to a number of poor health outcomes, including heart conditions. Excessive alcohol intake can lead to high blood pressure, heart failure or stroke. Excessive drinking can also contribute to cardiomyopathy, a disorder that affects the heart muscle. What's more, alcohol can contribute to obesity and the long list of health problems that can go along with it, McEvoy says: "Alcohol is a source of excess calories and a cause of weight gain that can be harmful in the long term."[121]

As stated, Cannabis causes high blood pressure with *initial* use, after this, it causes low blood pressure, and vasodilation—which are both good for the heart. Alcohol causes high blood pressure with excessive use. It can weaken the heart muscle, and cause a stroke. The warnings in the media are bias against cannabis, because alcohol is also a major culprit.

A "National Threat"

Despite the damage alcohol does to society, the Trump Administration singles out cannabis as a *national threat*. In the *Surgeon General's warning*, we read:

> *"This advisory is intended to raise awareness of the known and potential harms to developing brains, posed by the increasing availability of highly potent marijuana in multiple, concentrated forms. These harms are costly to individuals and to our society, impacting mental health and educational achievement and raising the risks of addiction and misuse of other substances."*

---

120 *Increased Blood Pressure Following Abrupt Cessation of Daily Cannabis Use*. JOURNAL OF ADDICTION MEDICINE. PUB MED. March 6, 2011

121 *Alcohol and Heart Health: Separating Fact from Fiction*. JOHNS HOPKINS

The Surgeon General warns us about the effect cannabis has on "developing brains." First of all, no one advocates allowing children to consume cannabis. No one over 21 can buy cannabis legally at a recreational dispensary. Secondly, alcohol causes far greater damage. We read:

> "Consuming alcohol significantly alters mood, behavior, and neuropsychological functioning. That's why many people turn to alcohol as a way to relax, escape, or socialize. But drinking while underage can cause significant developmental problems. Due to the fact that their brain and other organs are still developing, adolescents are more susceptible to becoming dependent. This dependency raises the chances of teen alcohol poisoning."[122]

Brain damage caused by alcohol has been confirmed in brain scans. From *NPR*, we read:

> "A recent study led by neuroscientist Susan Tapert of the University of California, San Diego compared the brain scans of teens who drink heavily with the scans of teens who don't. Tapert's team found damaged nerve tissue in the brains of the teens who drank. The researchers believe this damage negatively affects attention span in boys, and girls' ability to comprehend and interpret visual information."[123]

We are warned about the impact cannabis has on "educational achievement." Of course. Any substance that intoxicates will have a negative impact on learning, including Alcohol:

> "Alcohol consumption showed negative associations with motivation for and subjectively achieved academic performance. University alcohol prevention activities might have positive impact on students' academic success."[124]

If "low educational outcomes" is the standard for making *any* substance illegal, alcohol should also be banned. This is no reason to keep responsible *adults* from cannabis. Especially, if they need it medicinally.

The Surgeon General continues with this warning:

> *"Additionally, marijuana use remains illegal for youth under state law in all states; normalization of its use raises the*

122 **The Scary Truth About Teen Alcohol Poisoning**. NEWPORT ACADEMY

123 **Teen Drinking May Cause Irreversible Brain Damage**. NPR CPR News. January 25, 2010

124 **Is Alcohol Consumption Associated with Poor Academic Achievement in University Students?** PUBMED. October4, 2013

potential for criminal consequences in this population. In addition to the health risks posed by marijuana use, sale or possession of marijuana remains illegal under federal law notwithstanding some state laws to the contrary."

This warning is a reason to legalize the drug. Who want's a prison sentence to ruin a young adult's life, for a drug safer than alcohol? President Trump supports current laws, and regulations that send these people to prison, causing them to choose a life of crime, because prison records affect chances of employment.

Pregnant Women

The Surgeon General continues by giving a warning to pregnant women about cannabis use:

""Pregnant women use marijuana more than any other illicit drug. In a national survey, marijuana use in the past month among pregnant women doubled (3.4% to 7%) between 2002 and 201712. In a study conducted in a large health system, marijuana use rose by 69% (4.2% to 7.1%) between 2009 and 2016 among pregnant women13. Alarmingly, many retail dispensaries recommend marijuana to pregnant women for morning sickness14. Marijuana use during pregnancy can affect the developing fetus. THC can enter the fetal brain from the mother's bloodstream. It may disrupt the endocannabinoid system, which is important for a healthy pregnancy and fetal brain development1 Studies have shown that marijuana use in pregnancy is associated with adverse outcomes, including lower birth weight15. The Colorado Pregnancy Risk Assessment Monitoring System reported that maternal marijuana use was associated with a 50% increased risk of low birth weight regardless of maternal age, race, ethnicity, education, and tobacco use16. The American College of Obstetricians and Gynecologists holds that "[w]omen who are pregnant or contemplating pregnancy should be encouraged to discontinue marijuana use. Women reporting marijuana use should be counseled about concerns regarding potential adverse health consequences of continued use during pregnancy"17. In 2018, the American Academy of Pediatrics recommended that "... it is important to advise all adolescents and young women that if they become pregnant, marijuana should not be used during pregnancy"

Certainly, pregnant women should not use cannabis. And, despite the fact that using cannabis during pregnancy can cause low birth weight in about

50 percent of users, it is not significant. From MD Edge, we read:

> "The effects are unclear. Marijuana use during pregnancy is associated with clinically unimportant lower birth weights (growth differences of approximately 100 g), but no differences in preterm births or congenital anomalies (strength of recommendation [SOR]:B, prospective and retrospective cohort studies with methodologic flaws)."[125]

According to these physicians, low birth weight caused by Cannabis is "clinically unimportant." Not only this, but the statement itself needs some perspective. Caffeine use during pregnancy can also cause low birth weight. From Web Md, we read:

> "New research suggests that caffeine is linked to low-birth-weight babies and that drinking coffee is linked to a longer pregnancy. The report suggests that drinking 200-300 milligrams of caffeine per day raised the risk of a baby being born small by between 27% and 62%. Smaller babies have higher risks of certain health problems, and the researchers say recommendations on safe limits need to be reconsidered."[126]

Caffeine in coffee, tea, and energy drinks can cause low birth weights up to 62%. With cannabis, it is up to 50%. The percentage of women who experience this is not the issue—but *how much* weight does it cause the baby to lose? If "statistically insignificant," this is no cause for alarm.

The news reports touted this percentage trying to damage the cannabis legalization movement. This does not mean cannabis use during pregnancy is safe. Studies are not complete, and there could be unseen effects. At this point, we don't know. And, it is probably not safe to use *any drug* during pregnancy. Alcohol is legal, and can cause "fetal alcohol syndrome." From *Alcohol and Drug Research*, we read:

> "Exposure to alcohol during development produces Fetal Alcohol Spectrum Disorders (FASD), characterized by a wide range of effects that include deficits in multiple cognitive domains. Early identification and treatment of individuals with FASD remains a challenge because neurobehavioral alterations do not become a significant problem until late childhood and early adolescence. ...Together these data suggest that moderate prenatal alcohol exposure alters the disinhibitory function in the OFC, which may contribute to the executive function deficits associated with

125 *Clinical Inquiries. What Effects—if any—does marijuana Use During Pregnancy Have on the Fetus or Child?* MD EDGE. July, 2017

126 *Caffeine Linked to Low-Birth-Weight Babies*. WEB MD. February 19, 2019

FASD."[127]

As with cannabis hyperemesis syndrome, mitochondrial dysfunction can also contribute to low birth weights. A recent study of piglets demonstrated a direct relationship. From Oxidative Medicine, and Cellular Longevity, we read:

> "Intrauterine growth restriction (IUGR) is associated with fetal mortality and morbidity. One of the most common causes of IUGR is placental insufficiency, including placental vascular defects, and mitochondrial dysfunction. In addition, a high level of oxidative stress induces placental vascular lesions. Here, we evaluated the oxidative stress status, mitochondrial function, angiogenesis, and nutrient transporters in placentae of piglets with different birth weights... Collectively, placentae for lower birth weight neonates are vulnerable to oxidative damage, mitochondrial dysfunction, and impaired angiogenesis."[128]

If a woman suffers from mitochondrial dysfunction, the same genetic condition that could trigger CHS also can cause low birth weights *without* cannabis use. However, if someone with this genetic condition uses cannabis, the risk of a low birth weight could be greater. The same is true for any substance that has a negative impact on the mitochondria. Opiates also cause mitochondria dysfunction. From Anesthesiology, we read:

> "Although the extent to which they alter mitochondrial function in vivo is not yet understood, it has long been known that intravenous drugs with anesthetic properties can depress carbohydrate metabolism, oxygen consumption, and energy production in the nervous system. Early studies of narcotics demonstrated that they inhibit oxidation of glucose, lactate, and pyruvate in neural tissues at clinically relevant concentrations, and seven decades later, it has been proposed that morphine may actually have a mitochondrial-based mechanism of clinical action. ...The primary effect of barbiturates on oxidative phosphorylation in mitochondria obtained from brain, heart, and liver also seems to be inhibition of complex I, and, like propofol, they seem to "uncouple" metabolic activity from ATP production, further reducing bioenergetic capacity."[129]

127 *Moderate prenatal alcohol exposure alters the number and function of GABAergic interneurons in the murine orbitofrontal cortex* ALCOHOL AND DRUG RESEARCH. PUB MED June 12, 2020

128 *Placentae for Low Birth Weight Piglets Are Vulnerable to Oxidative Stress, Mitochondrial Dysfunction, and Impaired Angiogenesis*. Oxidative medicine and cellular longevity. OXIDATIVE MEDICINE AND CELLULAR LONGEVITY. PUB MED. May 25, 2020

129 *Clinical Implications of Mitochondrial Dysfunction*. ANESTHESIOLOGY. October 2006

Opiates, which include morphine, cause mitochondrial dysfunction. Opiates also cause low birth weight. We read:

> "Infants born to opiate-dependent women frequently have low birth weights and low 1- and 5-min Apgar scores. Significant postnatal problems, excluding neonatal withdrawal, can include jaundice, infection, aspiration pneumonia, transient tachypnea, and hyaline membrane disease. Neonatal abstinence may be severe and persist for as long as 3 months. Abstinence symptoms can include central nervous system hyperirritability, gastrointestinal dysfunction, respiratory distress, tremors, fever, high-pitched cry, increased muscle tone, uncoordinated sucking and swallowing reflexes, dehydration, and possible electrolyte imbalance. During the first week of life, increased respirations associated with hypocapnia and alkalosis may occur. The Brazelton Neonatal Behavioral Assessment Scale has been used to quantify the neurobehavioral effects on neonates of narcotics administered prenatally. A marked decline in mortality rates of infants born to opiate-dependent mothers is evident."[130]

Opiates also cause low birth weights, and mitochondrial dysfunction, the same as cannabis. Only opiates cause many other serious issues, such as jaundice, infection, and aspiration pneumonia. It is hypocritical to use "low birth weights" as an excuse to continue cannabis prohibition, when opiates cause more problems for the baby.

The Surgeon General continues:

> *"Maternal marijuana use may still be dangerous to the baby after birth. THC has been found in breast milk for up to six days after the last recorded use. It may affect the newborn's brain development and result in hyperactivity, poor cognitive function, and other long-term consequences. Additionally, marijuana smoke contains many of the same harmful components as tobacco smoke. No one should smoke marijuana or tobacco around a baby."*

Why be so concerned with THC in breast milk, but not opiates, or alcohol? The Surgeon General repeats an old assumption, that has never been proven. From *Pediatrics*, we read:

> "There are limited data on the potential neurobehavioral effects of infant exposure to cannabis through breast milk. Astley and

---

130 *Effects of maternal opiate abuse on the newborn.* FEDERATION PROCEEDINGS. PUBMED. April, 1995

Little reported psychomotor deficits in fifty five 12-month-old infants breastfed by mothers using cannabis compared with 81 unexposed infants. In contrast, Tennes et al reported no differences in motor and mental development in twenty seven 12-month-old infants whose mothers used marijuana while breastfeeding compared with 35 unexposed infants."[131]

These "facts" posted by the Surgeon General are designed to scare the average citizen into supporting cannabis prohibition. If cannabis *did* cause low educational outcomes, hyperactivity, and brain damage in children, we would be warned that *"will all live in a world of criminals, and leeches on society."* That is the alarmist tone behind these words. Instead, alcohol has been linked to low educational outcomes, and brain damage, and everyone can observe it's negative impact society.

Cannabis and Autism Rates

It is also curious the Surgeon General did not post any warnings about a potential link between autism, and cannabis use during pregnancy. Since this has been on the news lately, it would no doubt also be part of a future White House campaign against cannabis. *Forbes* reported:

"Researchers from The Ottawa Hospital and affiliated institutions reviewed data from every birth in Ontario, Canada, between 2007 and 2012, which summed up to more than 500,000, in what is believed to be one of the most extensive studies of its kind. In 2,200 cases the mothers said they used marijuana during pregnancy without mixing it with tobacco, alcohol or opioids. The study found "an association between maternal cannabis use in pregnancy and the incidence of autism spectrum disorder in the offspring." "The incidence of autism spectrum disorder diagnosis was 4.00 per 1,000 person-years among children with exposure compared to 2.42 among unexposed children, and the fully adjusted hazard ratio was 1.51," according to the study."[132]

I want to reiterate that *no drugs* should be used during pregnancy, including cannabis. At this point, we do not know the risks. Yet, this study—although more extensive than many others— has flaws for several reasons. First, it uses "self-reporting" of cannabis use. We read again from *Forbes*:

"The authors of the Canadian study published Thursday acknowledged that it is limited. It did not capture the amount and

131 *Marijuana Use by Breastfeeding Mothers and Cannabinoid Concentrations in Breast Milk.* PEDIATRICS. PUBMED. August 21, 2018

132 *Marijuana Use During Pregnancy Linked To Autism In Children: Study*. FORBES. August 10, 2020

type of marijuana the women used or when during the pregnancy or how often women used it."

This study admits it did *not* factor "when during pregnancy or how often women used it." Yet, consider how this could be used by an anti-cannabis activists who run the White House. If they could get you to believe cannabis causes autism among the general population, you would likely not object to a industry shutdown.

This would not be based on facts, because it is much more complex. Cannabis use by itself doesn't cause autism, but combined with other substances, and when there is a mutation in the Mitochondrial DNA, it almost certainly contributes.

This study separated mothers who used cannabis alone, from those who used cannabis with opiates. And, for good reason. Opiates also increase the risk of autism. From the Centers for Disease Control, we read:

> "A study from the Waisman Center at the University of Wisconsin-Madison, in collaboration with the Centers for Disease Control and Prevention (CDC), found that mothers who were prescribed opioids just before becoming pregnant were more likely to have a child with autism spectrum disorder (ASD) or a child with other developmental disabilities (DDs) and some autism symptoms. This study is among the first to look at associations between prescription of opioids in pregnancy and ASD and other DDs. More research is needed to better understand developmental outcomes among children whose mothers used opioids before (meaning 3 months before) and during pregnancy."[133]

As Cannabis, Opiates also cause a mitochondrial pathology. From Anesthesiology, we read:

> "Although the extent to which they alter mitochondrial function in vivo is not yet understood, it has long been known that intravenous drugs with anesthetic properties can depress carbohydrate metabolism, oxygen consumption, and energy production in the nervous system. Early studies of narcotics demonstrated that they inhibit oxidation of glucose, lactate, and pyruvate in neural tissues at clinically relevant concentrations, and seven decades later, it has been proposed that morphine may actually have a mitochondrial-based mechanism of clinical action."[134]

Opiate addicts have aberrant, altered mitochondria DNA. We read:

133 *Key Findings: Opioids Prescribed Just Before Pregnancy Associated With Autism*. CDC
134 *Clinical Implications of Mitochondrial Dysfunction*. ANESTHESIOLOGY. October 2006

"Because mitochondrial abnormalities have been associated with opiate addiction, we examined the effect of morphine on mtDNA levels in rat and mouse models of addiction and in cultured cells. We found that mtDNA copy number was significantly reduced in the hippocampus and peripheral blood of morphine-addicted rats and mice compared with control animals."[135]

The Surgeon General goes into great detail warning about the effects of THC on the cannabinoid receptors, but opiates act on opiate receptors, and change DNA. It has a worse effect on the mitochondria, although the risk of autism is increased with the use of almost any drug. But these drugs appear to be a secondary cause.

Pregnant women who suffer from a specific illness have even a higher risk of giving birth to an autistic child. From *Science Daily*, we read:

"Children whose mothers had hyperemesis gravidarum -- a severe form of a morning sickness -- during pregnancy were 53% more likely to be diagnosed with autism spectrum disorder, according to Kaiser Permanente research published in the American Journal of Perinatology. "This study is important because it suggests that children born to women with hyperemesis may be at an increased risk of autism," said lead study author Darios Getahun, MD, PhD, of Kaiser Permanente Southern California Department of Research and Evaluation. "Awareness of this association may create the opportunity for earlier diagnosis and intervention in children at risk of autism." Hyperemesis gravidarum occurs in less than 5% of pregnancies. Affected women experience intense nausea and are unable to keep down food and fluids. This can lead to dangerous dehydration and inadequate nutrition during pregnancy. To determine the extent of the association between hyperemesis gravidarum and autism spectrum disorder, researchers reviewed electronic health records of nearly 500,000 pregnant women and their children born between 1991 and 2014 at Kaiser Permanente in Southern California. They compared children whose mothers had a diagnosis of hyperemesis gravidarum during pregnancy to those whose mothers did not. Other findings from the research included:
• Exposure to hyperemesis gravidarum was associated with increased risk of autism when hyperemesis gravidarum was diagnosed during the first and second trimesters of pregnancy, but not when it was diagnosed only in the third trimester.
• Exposure to hyperemesis gravidarum was associated with risk

---

135 *Decreased mitochondrial DNA copy number in the hippocampus and peripheral blood during opiate addiction is mediated by autophagy and can be salvaged by melatonin*. TAYLOR FRANCIS ONLINE. September 30, 2012

of autism regardless of the severity of the mother's hyperemesis gravidarum.

• The association between hyperemesis gravidarum and autism spectrum disorder was stronger in girls than boys and among whites and Hispanics than among blacks and Pacific Islanders.

• The medications used to treat hyperemesis gravidarum did not appear to be related to autism risk.

The results are consistent with the hypothesis that women experiencing hyperemesis gravidarum have poor nutritional intake, which may, in turn lead to potential long-term neurodevelopment impairment in their children. The study cannot, however, rule out other possible explanations, such as perinatal exposures to some medications and maternal smoking."[136]

As hyperemesis gravidarum rises the risk of autism, autistic children have been found to have a disruption in their mitochondria:

"Children with autism are far more likely to have deficits in their ability to produce cellular energy than are typically developing children, a new study by researchers at UC Davis has found. The study, published in the Journal of the American Medical Association (JAMA), found that cumulative damage and oxidative stress in mitochondria, the cell's energy producer, could influence both the onset and severity of autism, suggesting a strong link between autism and mitochondrial defects." (Children with autism have mitochondrial dysfunction, study finds. SCIENCE DAILY. November 30, 2010[137])

Subsequent studies have demonstrated that mitochondrial dysfunction can cause several complications during pregnancy, including cognitive defects. From *Mitochondrial Disease News*, we read:

"Women with mitochondrial disease or mitochondrial dysfunction are more susceptible to complications during pregnancy, and their newborns are more likely to have congenital defects, a retrospective study shows. The study, " Effects of mitochondrial disease/disfunction on pregnacy: A retrospective study," was published in Mitochondrion. Primary mitochondrial disease (MD) comprises several rare disorders caused by genetic mutations in nuclear and mitochondrial DNA,

---

136 *Severe morning sickness associated with higher risk of autism.*
SCIENCE DAILY. October 3, 2019
137 *Children with autism have mitochondrial dysfunction, study finds.*
SCIENCE DAILY. November 30, 2010

whereas mitochondrial dysfunction (Md) may develop through environmental exposure, medications, infection or other non-genetic factors. Both MD and Md lead to mitochondria malfunction, in particular decreased production of adenosine triphosphate (ATP) — the energy molecule used by all cells in the body— by the mitochondrial respiratory chain (MRC), which has a direct impact on cell function. During pregnancy, metabolic demands increase to allow fetal development and growth, which requires optimal and efficient energy production."[138]

Let's connect these facts. (1) It is known that mitochondrial dysfunction can cause problems during pregnancy. (2) Scientists believe this disease is genetic, but could potentially be caused by other factors, including the environment, medications, and infection. (3) Mitochondrial dysfunction has been linked to "cyclic vomiting syndrome." (4) Women who suffer from Hyperemesis gravidarum likely also suffer from it. (5) Autistic children have a dysfunction in their mitochondria. (6) Opiates, cannabis, and other drugs can further mitochondrial dysfunction. The connections are obvious. And other factors have been linked to a rise in autism rates. In *Spectrum News*, we read:

"For a pregnant woman, the factors that can raise autism risk in her unborn child may seem to abound. Studies suggest that getting the flu, having a fever or gaining too much weight while pregnant can all boost the odds of having a child with autism. Certain medications may also raise the risk. For instance, pregnant women who take the epilepsy drug valproate are up to seven times more likely to have a child with autism than those who don't. In the past three months, studies have linked three more types of pills to autism risk: antidepressants, acetaminophen and a class of asthma drugs. Mothers-to-be who take these drugs may as much as double their risk of having a child with autism. Still, the absolute risk of autism remains small — an important point that sometimes gets lost in the alarmist media coverage of these studies. Going off necessary medications can be risky, too. That's why some experts are urging caution in interpreting the results. "An important issue to keep in mind is that these are indeed large epidemiological studies, and the application of those findings to an individual is going to be more complex," says Geraldine Dawson, director of the Duke Center for Autism and Brain Development at Duke University in Durham, North Carolina." [139]

138 *Women with Mitochondrial Disease More Prone to Pregnancy Complications, Study Shows.* MITOCHONDRIAL DISEASE NEWS. August 10, 2018

139 *Taking meds during pregnancy brings autism risk, benefits.* SPECTRUM NEWS. By Emily Amthes. March 10, 2016

The "benefits" of taking some medications during autism, according to this article, would be the treatment of epilepsy. The epilepsy drug valproate raises the risk of autism by *seven times*. Cannabis treats epilepsy, but doesn't raise the risk anywhere near this. Therefore, it would be a safer medication for pregnant epileptics to use. And in both cases, it likely raises the risk among people who a mutation in the mitochondrial DNA.

Marijuana Use during Adolescence

The Surgeon General Continues:

"Marijuana is also commonly used by adolescents, second only to alcohol. In 2017, approximately 9.2 million youth aged 12 to 25 reported marijuana use in the past month and 29% more young adults aged 18-25 started using marijuana. In addition, high school students' perception of the harm from regular marijuana use has been steadily declining over the last decade. During this same period, a number of states have legalized adult use of marijuana for medicinal or recreational purposes, while it remains illegal under federal law. The legalization movement may be impacting youth perception of harm from marijuana."

There is *one* fact in this statement: more kids use alcohol than cannabis. Alcohol causes learning problems, and sometimes death. The decline in the perceived harm in marijuana among our youth is based on *science*, not legalization. For years, scare tactics full of errors were taught to our children. Now we have the internet, and these lies can no longer exist in a vacuum. Furthermore, cannabis use among young people has declined in legal cannabis states. We read:

"More teens are choosing not to use marijuana, according to new survey results from the City and County of Denver. The city believes its new "facts-based" marijuana youth prevention campaign is part of the reason for the improving stats. Denver's "High Costs marijuana youth education and prevention campaign," or just High Costs, is an effort by the City and County of Denver to educate Denver's youth on how underage marijuana-use can affect their passions, pursuits and futures. Instead of promoting scare tactics, Denver's campaign focuses on providing facts for teens, so they can have accurate peer-to-peer conversations. But education has not always been the main goal of drug prevention campaigns in the past." [140]

Drug education based on truth, and responsibility works. The federal

140 ***Study finds more teens are choosing not to use marijuana***. 9 NEWS. February 29, 2020

government on the other hand, has caused kids not to trust adults on this issue. When it makes such a big deal about marijuana, and treats it worse than booze, kids pay attention. They know that booze is worse than pot. So when people in our the government state the opposite, they don't believe true information about really bad drugs.

As stated, when cannabis is sold legally in stores to adults, less is sold in the black market, and kids have less access. The Trump Administration is so concerned with legalization "sending the wrong idea" to kids, they ignore the really bad drug, alcohol. Are they concerned enough to stop beer advertisements on television? Are they concerned with the message legal beer sales in grocery stores send to our children? No. To them, booze as a legitimate industry, not cannabis. President Trump has it backwards. Alcohol is far worse.

The legalization of cannabis for adults has changed the conversation for the better. Instead of teaching kids that no one should ever do it, they are taught to wait until they are adults, after the brain is fully developed. This approach has worked in the city of Denver.

One physician was asked which drug he would rather his child do, alcohol or cannabis. Here is his response, in an opinion piece in the New York Times:

> "As my children, and my friends' children, are getting older, a question that comes up again and again from friends is this: Which would I rather my children use — alcohol or marijuana? The immediate answer, of course, is "neither."...I've seen young people brought to the emergency room because they've consumed too much alcohol and become poisoned. That happens thousands of times a year. Some even die...When someone asks me whether I'd rather my children use pot or alcohol, after sifting through all the studies and all the data, I still say "neither." Usually, I say it more than once. But if I'm forced to make a choice, the answer is "marijuana."[141]

Instead of the Trump Administration afraid that the legalization of cannabis will cause youth to perceive it to be safe, he should be concerned that legal sales of alcohol make it appear safer. Every year, kids die from alcohol poisoning. They are receiving the wrong message from the federal government. The Surgeon General continues:

> *"The human brain continues to develop from before birth into the mid-20s and is vulnerable to the effects of addictive substances. Frequent marijuana use during adolescence is associate with: Changes in the areas of the brain involved in attention, memory, decision-making, and motivation. Deficits in attention and memory have been detected in marijuana-using teens even after*

---

141 ***Alcohol or Marijuana? A Pediatrician Faces the Question*** By Aaron E. Carroll New York Times, March 16, 2015

a month of abstinence."

The claim that "Deficits in attention and memory have been detected in marijuana-using teens even a month of abstinence" footnotes to a study "Cannabis and alcohol use, and the developing brain." The study cited is *not* making this claim about cannabis only, but about cannabis *and alcohol*. But that is not what the reader assumes. The reader assumes that cannabis alone is causing a memory deficit that is permanent. But as we have already read, it is alcohol. Once again, the government attempts to trick the reader.

The Surgeon General continues warning about "declines in IQ":

> *"Impaired learning in adolescents. Chronic use is linked to declines in IQ, school performance that jeopardizes professional and social achievements, and life satisfaction."*

In the last chapter, I presented two studies that refuted this belief of the President's. One study tracked two sets of identical twins, another study tracked a large group of people over two decades, and no difference in IQ was noted. Since alcohol is socially acceptable, and legal, almost no child uses cannabis exclusively, without first drinking alcohol. And, it has been proven that alcohol lowers IQ's—not only in children, but also adults. After this, we read:

> *"Increased rates of school absence and drop-out, as well as suicide attempts."*

Many children that drop out of school have other issues at home, and these problems cause other drugs to be used, not only cannabis. Adolescents with these problems sometimes attempt suicide. Furthermore, these children suffer from a wide range of problems. Cannabis is one of many drugs, including alcohol, problem kids use as to escape.

No studies exist that directly link cannabis use to suicide attempts, and the study the Surgeon General cites only proves cannabis is a symptom of an underlying problem. After this, a "footnote trick" is again used. We read:

> *"Risk for and early onset of psychotic disorders, such as schizophrenia. The risk for psychotic disorders increases with frequency of use, potency of the marijuana product, and as the age at first use decreases."*

This claim was refuted in a previous chapter. The study cited as proof that cannabis rises "early onset of psychotic disorders, such as schizophrenia" used flawed methods. They did surveys of mental institutions, and calculated cannabis use. This is not a true representation of the population. However, the claim there is "risk for...early onset" of these disorders," with cannabis use, is likely true. Schizophrenia is a genetic condition, and schizophrenics suffer from higher dopamine levels. At first use, cannabis raises dopamine levels, and therefore could set off a latent condition. With use however, cannabis *blunts* dopamine response[142], and therefore could be a potential treatment.

After this, the Surgeon General blames cannabis for a rise in opiate abuse:

> *Other substance use. In 2017, teens 12-17 reporting frequent use of marijuana showed a 130% greater likelihood of misusing opioids.*

This statement is footnoted to the study **"Substance Abuse and Mental Health Services Administration. (2018). Key Substance Use and Mental Health Indicators in the United States: Results from the 2017 National Survey on Drug Use and Health."** This survey is a *national* survey, which means that it takes into account States that have not legalized cannabis. This skews the results. As proven in a previous chapter, states that legalized cannabis witnessed a decline in opiate use:

> "Eight studies reported associations between policies decriminalizing marijuana and reduced prescription opioid use, 1 study was inconclusive, and the retrospective cohort study reported an increase in adverse opioid-related outcomes. These results should be interpreted with caution given limitations associated with the studies' design. Results demonstrating association between marijuana decriminalization and opioid-related outcomes are mixed. Longitudinal studies are needed, and further analysis of this policy should continue to be tracked."[143]

Studies that looked specifically at states where recreational, or medical cannabis was legalized have witnessed a decline in opiate use. This "national survey" cited by the Surgeon General looks at national statistics. This presents a false picture. It does not prove "cannabis does something to the brain, that causes people to want to try opiates"—or similar rubbish. Instead, the overall national opiate epidemic is reflected in these statistics. What happened nationally? People in government took large sums of money from the pharmaceutical industry, and passed laws that allowed legal opiate sales to flourish. This is reflected in these national statistics, and has nothing to do with cannabis legalization. Both merely occurred at the same time.

After this, the Surgeon General concludes:

---

142 **The effects of Δ9-tetrahydrocannabinol on the dopamine system** NATURE. PUBMED. November 17, 2016

143 **Is There Less Opioid Abuse in States Where Marijuana Has Been Decriminalized, Either for Medicinal or Recreational Use? A Clin-IQ.** JOURNAL OF PATIENT-CENTERED RESEARCH AND REVIEWS. PUBMED. October 29, 2019

*"Marijuana's increasingly widespread availability in multiple
and highly potent forms, coupled with a false and dangerous
perception of safety among youth, merits a nationwide call to
action."*

The conclusion of the Surgeon General's warning calls for a "nationwide call to action." This is reminiscent of President Richard Nixon's rallying cry to the nation when he declared a "war on drugs." He called drug abuse "public enemy number one." The term "nationwide call to action" is similar to Nixon's call for support.

In the last State of the Union address, the main topic was opiate addiction. President Trump took credit for a reduction in opiate use, but in reality, several factors unrelated to any of his actions caused this decline—including cannabis reforms. If Trump is reelected, there is a good chance that an ad campaign will be produced, possibly funded by "anti-cannabis donors," including Smart Approaches to Marijuana. These ads will saturate the airways, and will blame cannabis for opiate addiction, schizophrenia, autism, and violence. Cannabis will be targeted as a "gateway drug." The President will ask the public for support, then instruct the FDA and IRS to begin levying fines on all dispensaries, which are breaking federal drug laws. This would eliminate profits, and put end the legal cannabis market.

CHAPTER 7
BEHIND THE SCENES

The sound bites of President Trump in support of legal cannabis have been embraced by his supporters, while multiple anti-cannabis actions have gone unnoticed. His support for reforms cannot be true, considering all of the facts. From the very beginning, President Trump has sought to retain his power to shut down cannabis dispensaries. The Cole Memorandum protected state marijuana businesses from Federal interference. This memo was rescinded by former Attorney General Jeff Sessions. From *Bank Law Monitor*, we read:

> "Reiterating that Congress considers marijuana to be a "dangerous drug" and marijuana activity to be a "serious crime," Attorney General Jeff Sessions today issued a memo to all U.S. attorneys rescinding various memoranda related to enforcement of federal marijuana laws issued during the Obama administration. Included in the rescinded memos was the prominent "Cole Memo," which discouraged federal prosecution of anyone in compliance with the marijuana laws of their state. As we previously discussed, the Cole Memo specifically provided the justification on which many banks and credit unions decided to offer financial services to marijuana and marijuana-related businesses. While the full effects of Sessions' memo remain unclear, today certainly appears to mark a shift in the federal government's stance on state-legalized marijuana, and the future of marijuana banking is as hazy as ever."[144]

---

144 *DOJ Rescinds the Cole Memo—What It Means for Your Financial Institution* BANK LAW MONITOR. By Kalin Bornemann and Danielle Hunt on January 4, 2018

After these actions, many believed the former Attorney General was acting rouge. We know now that this was not the case. President Trump assembled the *Marijuana Policy Coordination Committee*. The President also made statements in support of this action. As stated in a previous chapter, when he signed the budget, he stated three times that he retains the power to enforce all federal cannabis laws, despite a provision in these bills that protected States rights[145]. He has made this statement *every time* he signed the budget. Only he wants this protection to be ended, *in the year following his reelection*:

> "President Trump proposed ending an existing policy that protects state medical marijuana programs from Justice Department interference as part of his fiscal year 2021 budget plan released on Monday. The rider, which has been renewed in appropriations legislation every year since 2014, stipulates the Justice Department can't use its funds to prevent states or territories "from implementing their own laws that authorize the use, distribution, possession, or cultivation of medical marijuana." This isn't the first time that an administration has requested that the rider be stricken...When Trump signed that large-scale spending legislation in December, he attached a statement that said he is empowered to ignore the congressionally approved medical cannabis rider, stating that the administration "will treat this provision consistent with the President's constitutional responsibility to faithfully execute the laws of the United States."[146]

President Trump signed the bill with the cannabis protection rider included three times, albeit grudgingly. The memo circulated in the DEA reveals

---

145 "In a statement attached to a large-scale funding bill he signed into law on Friday, President Trump said in effect that he reserves the right to ignore a congressionally approved provision that seeks to protect state medical marijuana laws from federal interference. "Division B, section 531 of the Act provides that the Department of Justice may not use any funds made available under this Act to prevent implementation of medical marijuana laws by various States and territories," Trump wrote in a signing statement. "My Administration will treat this provision consistent with the President's constitutional responsibility to faithfully execute the laws of the United States." Although the vague language doesn't directly say he plans to ignore Congress's will to block Justice Department prosecution of medical cannabis patients and providers, presidents typically use signing statements such as this one to flag provisions of laws they are enacting which they believe could impede on their executive authorities. By calling out the medical marijuana rider, Trump is making clear that his administration believes it can broadly enforce federal drug laws against people complying with state medical marijuana laws even though Congress told him not to." ***Trump Says He Can Ignore Medical Marijuana Protections Passed By Congress***. By Tom Angell. FORBES. Dec 21, 2019

146 ***Trump Budget Proposes Ending State Medical Marijuana Protections And Blocking DC From Legalizing***. MARIJUANA MOMENT. February 10, 2020

why. His legal team instructed them to change their policies, to conform to international law. The Memo indicates the government must seize all crops, and form a monopoly. The rider in the bill could prevent all of this.

Negative Input

After the news of the President's *Marijuana Policy Coordination Committee* broke, their was a denial of any bias. President Trump claimed they were looking at both positive and negative information. The actions of the former Attorney General paint a different picture. As he was sitting in meetings of the "anti-cannabis cabinet," he had a meeting exclusively with these people, who are all against the cannabis industry:

> Edwin Meese III, Attorney General under the Reagan administration
> Kevin Sabet, president and CEO of Smart Approaches to Marijuana
> Bertha Madras, a former Office of National Drug Control Policy staffer and a member of President Trump's Commission on Combating Drug Addiction and the Opioid Crisis
> Robert DuPont, former director of the National Institute on Drug Abuse
> David Evans, executive director of the Drug Free Schools Coalition[147]

This meeting proves that President Trump is only concerned with negative information about cannabis. He sought out voices that echo his anti-cannabis views, including a former law enforcement official. A man who ran the drug war under Ronald Reagan. As President Trump's spokesman stated *"more enforcement is coming,"* the former Attorney General spoke similar words at this meeting:

> "I think it's a big issue for America, for the country, and I'm of the general view that this is not a healthy substance," Sessions said at the beginning of the gathering. "I think that's pretty clear. And then have the policy response that we and the federal government needs to be prepared to take and do so appropriately and with good sense."[148]

This "policy response" of the Federal government *is* the "greater enforcement" that is coming, and will occur if Donald Trump is reelected.

---

147 *Jeff Sessions Just Met with These Anti-Cannabis Activists*. MARIJUANA MOMENT. December 8, 2019.
148 *idib*

An Attempt to block Cannabis exports from Israel

President Trump promised to support medical cannabis "one hundred percent" when he ran for office. This must be a lie, considering the pressure he put on Prime Minister Netanyahu. From the *Jerusalem Post*, we read:

> "Report: Netanyahu nixes medical marijuana export because of Trump The prime minister said US President had called him and expressed his objection to pot exports. The industry was expected to earn Israel $1-4 billion a year. Prime Minister Benjamin Netanyahu said US President Donald Trump called and expressed his objection to Israeli exports of marijuana, an industry expected to earn the country between $1b. and $4b. a year." [149]

The President gave Netanyahu the same reason for halting these exports that he gave the DEA, and FDA. *International treaties* must be followed, and they do not allow cannabis exports. Instead of siding with people who need cannabis as a medicine, he sided with the "swamp" of the United Nations. The United Nations has a bigger swamp than the United States. It is many "swamps" combined.

Instead of being a leader, and leading a effort at the U.N. to change a bad treaty, he takes it upon himself to interfere in the affairs of an ally. If Israel violates that treaty, it is up to the UN to sanction them. Only a man who wholeheartedly is against cannabis would interfere in this manner. He has no problem threatening to defund the World Health Organization. But when it is in his best interest, the President almost considers United Nations treaties "divinely inspired." Fortunately, after Netanyahu agreed to obey Trump's wishes, the Knesset voted to allow these cannabis exports anyway.

Will Not Support Cannabis Business During Pandemic

President Trump has no problem giving pandemic relief to alcohol companies, but not dispensaries:

> "The cannabis lobby is flexing its muscle in Washington and seeking aid for small businesses in the next coronavirus relief package... But the push for help from Washington, where the federal government still classifies marijuana as a controlled substance, has so far failed to make headway...The GOP-controlled Senate will be a harder sell. In 2019, marijuana business advocates had high hopes for passing legislation that would allow financial institutions to finally do business with cannabis businesses that were legal in the states. The House passed legislation in

149 *Report: Netanyahu nixes medical marijuana export because of Trump*. JERUSALEM POST. February 7, 2018

September that would allow banks to finally work with cannabis businesses, but the bill failed to move in the Senate."[150]

How can President Trump be for medical "one hundred percent," and not help *medical* cannabis dispensaries in this time of crisis? Medicine is essential. This illustrates how much President Trump is against this industry. He also refuses to let cannabis businesses access banking. How is it possible to take these positions, and also support reforms?

The Trump Administration Blackmailed Schools Over Medical Cannabis

Although only one out of a thousand epilepsy patients die of their seizures, they are debilitating, even if deaths do not occur. One cannabinoid drug has been approved by the government for these seizures—Epidiolex. It uses a CBD distillate.

Any epileptic could die of their seizures at any time. Recently, a child star on the Disney Channel died. From *WebMd*, we read:

> "Disney Channel star Cameron Boyce died from a seizure Saturday at age 20. On Tuesday, his family released a statement that the actor had been treated for epilepsy, ABC News reports...Epilepsy is a common neurological disorder, the hallmark of which is unprovoked seizures. It affects people of all ages, though it's more common among young children and older people."[151]

Seizures can kill epileptics, or damage them permanently. As stated previously, though CBD has proven to be a miraculous treatment, there are some forms of epilepsy that only respond to a CBD/THC combination:

> "Both Δ9 Tetrahydrocannabidiol (THC) and cannabidiol (CBD) components of cannabis, have been shown to have anticonvulsant effects. Cannabis oils are used to treat seizures in drug-resistant epilepsy (DRE). Recent trials provide data on dosing, side effects, and efficacy of CBD, yet there is a paucity of information on THC in epilepsy. Primary objective was to establish dosing and tolerability of TIL-TC150 - a cannabis plant extract produced by Tilray®, containing 100 mg/mL CBD and 2 mg/mL THC- in children with Dravet syndrome. Secondary objectives were to assess impact of therapy on seizures, ...Twenty children received add-on therapy with TIL-TC150. The dose ranged from 2 to 16 mg/kg/day of CBD and 0.04 to 0.32 mg/kg/day of THC. Patients were monitored for tolerability and adverse events, and secondary objectives... Nineteen participants completed the 20-week intervention. Mean

150 *Marijuana lobby presses for coronavirus relief funds*. THE HILL. April 15, 2020
151 *When Epilepsy is Fatal*. WEBMD. July 10, 2019

dose achieved was 13.3 mg/kg/day of CBD (range 7–16 mg/kg/day) and 0.27 mg/kg/day of THC (range 0.14–0.32 mg/kg/day). Adverse events, common during titration included somnolence, anorexia, and diarrhea. Abnormalities of liver transaminases and platelets were observed with concomitant valproic acid therapy. There was a statistically significant improvement in quality of life, reduction in EEG spike activity, and median motor seizure reduction of 70.6%, with 50% responder rate of 63%."[152]

Studies like this one should convince anyone that medical cannabis should be allowed at school. The life of any child is not more important than the "perception" this might have on the legalization movement. At the same time, suicide is the second leading cause of death among teenagers. President Trump wants schools to choose between epileptics who use cannabis, and kids that are depressed. For the sole purpose of trying to curtail legalization, the Administration has withheld funds from schools that administer medical cannabis:

> "A 2019 JAMA Pediatrics analysis found that more than 1 in 4 Maine children were diagnosed with at least one mental disorder, the highest rate in the country. The state's Department of Education announced earlier this month that the federal government will cut off funding dedicated to youth mental health program because of Maine's medical marijuana policy. In 2018, Maine won a five-year federal grant designed to boost social service infrastructures supporting student mental health. The grant provided the program, called Maine-AWARE, $1.1 million in annual funding. Maine received $2.2 million in the past two years and spent the money appropriately. According to the Lewiston Sun Journal, the feds informed the state's Education Department the rest of the funding will now be cut off. As Maine's state commissioner of education Pender Makin wrote in an email, state law allows students to consume medical marijuana on campus if they have a medical prescription. Other states with legal medical cannabis feature similar rules. Typically, these programs, including Maine's, exclude the use of smokable marijuana."[153]

Because a *few* children have notes from their doctors to use medical cannabis at school, the Trump Administration has withheld funds from *all* mentally depressed children. In my opinion, it is sick to turn you back on the mental health of hundreds of kids, only to achieve a political agenda. Trump

---

152 ***A prospective open-label trial of a CBD/THC cannabis oil in dravet syndrome*** ANNALS OF CLINICAL AND TRANSLATIONAL NEUROLOGY. PUBMED September 5, 2018
153 ***Feds To Withdraw Mental Health Grants From Schools Allowing Medical Marijuana*** THE FRESH TOAST May 18, 2020

cannot possibly support medical "one hundred percent," and be in favor of this action. The letter of the law is being used subtlety to move against all aspects of the cannabis industry, short of shutting it down. This cannot happen until after his reelection, or he would lose—and he knows it.

Immigrants are Immoral Who Use It

The hopes and dreams of a person who wants to immigrate into this country can be dashed in pieces, thanks to the cannabis policies of Donald Trump. It is unthinkable that a medical condition could disqualify a person for legal immigrant status, but it can if a person want's to treat it with cannabis. According to President Trump, these people are "morally unfit." In the *Fresh Toast*, we read:

> "A federal immigration agency claried on Friday that using marijuana or engaging in cannabis-related "activities" such as working for a dispensary—even in states where it's legal— is an immoral offense that makes immigrants ineligible for citizenship. When applying for naturalization, the process of gaining citizenship, individuals must have established "good moral character" in the years preceding the application. Good moral character is a vague requirement that has been criticized by scholars and civil rights advocates, as assessing morality is arguably subjective. According to the U.S. Citizenship and Immigration Services (USCIS), state-legal marijuana consumption renders individuals morally unfit for citizenship. The new policy clarication reects a sentiment once expressed by former Attorney General Jeff Sessions, who said that "good people don't smoke marijuana."" [154]

This belief—that smoking marijuana is morally unacceptable in all circumstances—is out of step with the American people. According to Gallop:

> "The poll released on Tuesday shows a continuation of the growing acceptance of cannabis use among Americans as more states opt to legalize marijuana for medical or recreational purposes. Seven-out-of-ten respondents said using cannabis is morally acceptable. Only 28 percent said the activity is morally unacceptable."[155]

Thousands of people use Cannabis for serious medical conditions.

154 *State-Legal Marijuana Use Makes Immigrants Morally Unfit for Citizenship, Trump Administration Warns* THE FRESH TOAST. April 19, 2019
155 *Marijuana Use Is More Moral Than Porn, Gay Relations and Wearing Animal Fur, Americans Say.* MARIJUANA MOMENT. June 23, 2020

President Trump has instructed border guards to disqualify any immigrant *for life* if they have used cannabis. He believes they are "morally unfit," to enter into this country. He needs to walk a mile in their slippers. Treating a medical condition with a plant God created is not immoral. What is immoral is *anger—* not in short supply at the White House these days.

Canadian Investors Banned for Life

The Trump Administration banned cannabis users because they are "immoral." He also has banned investors from Canada, and anyone who has anything to do with the Cannabis industry. From *Politico*, we read:

> "Canadians who work in the marijuana industry — and those who invest in the booming pot sector — risk a lifetime ban on travel to the U.S., according to a senior official overseeing US border operations. As Canada prepares to become the world's only major industrialized nation to legalize retail marijuana sales starting Oct. 17, the Canadian cannabis sector is projected to generate billions of dollars of revenue in coming years and Canadians have flocked to take jobs and buy stocks in the burgeoning industry. But the move has potential to disrupt border crossings between the U.S. and Canada for travelers who run afoul of American drug laws, even if their activities are legal in Canada."[156]

As stated in the DEA memo, President Trump believes investment in opium stocks should be permitted, but not investment in cannabis stocks. It is in this context that we can understand these actions. Restrictions like these were never imposed before, based solely on interviews. Of course, if a Canadian had a cannabis conviction on his record, he would be denied entrance into this country. But these guidelines were recently strengthened by this Administration, after cannabis was legalized in Canada.

After this report, the policy was softened a little. In these new instructions, Canadians who admit cannabis use will lose their Nexus pass, but be "technically admissible." From Global News, we read:

> "Cannabis use may be legal in Canada, but if U.S. border guards find out about it, a person could have their Nexus pass taken away or not granted in the first place, secret instructions issued to managers at U.S. border posts say. "If an alien admits to the use of marijuana (post legalization) he or she is technically admissible to the U.S., but would not be eligible for a Trusted Traveller Program," the instructions say. The instructions were intended only for supervisors at U.S. border posts and weren't supposed

---

156 ***U.S. official: Canadian marijuana users, workers and investors risk lifetime border ban.*** POLITICO. September 9, 2018

to be circulated below their rank level. Lower-level border officers got much simpler material." [157]

The "Nexus pass" allows people who have been prescreened to enter the country quicker. So, if someone admits cannabis use, passes will be taken away or not granted. But they will be "technically admissible." All this means is that government can still deny them entrance, but this glaring, blatant anti-cannabis action is softened a little in the regulations.

The fact that the Trump Administration would take this action in the first place demonstrates a hostility towards cannabis industry. There is no way he could truthfully support reforms, and take these actions.

The Administration is using the IRS Against Dispensaries

How could Donald Trump support medical cannabis "one hundred percent," yet selectively go after a dispensary, using the IRS? Democrats were threatening to impeach Attorney General William Barr for going after a dispensary, after he signed a pledge to respect States rights on this issue. During his confirmation hearing Barr said:

> "However, we either should have a federal law that prohibits marijuana everywhere, which I would support myself because I think it's a mistake to back off marijuana. However, if we want a federal approach—if we want states to have their own laws—then let's get there and get there in the right way."[158]

These words were similar to Jeff Sessions promise. He said federal law should be followed, or congress should change the law. However, Attorney General Barr apparently broke his promise. From the San Francisco Chronicle, we read:

> "Cannabis may be legal in California, but in the eyes of the federal government, a business selling it is just "a giant drug trafficker." At least that's what U.S. Tax Court Judge Mark Holmes of Washington, D.C., said in the case of Oakland's Harborside, one of the country's oldest and largest dispensaries, as the company tries to figure out how much it should pay in taxes. Nearly two years after legalization in California, cannabis businesses still face costly hurdles because of federal law that criminalizes marijuana possession, use and cultivation. Companies can't deduct all their business expenses on tax returns, and some can't use mainstream banks, resorting instead to credit unions or even armored trucks

157 *Canadians can lose Nexus passes over legal cannabis use in Canada: U.S. document* GLOBAL NEWS. February 20, 2020

158 *William Barr Says He Supports Federal Law Prohibiting Marijuana Across the U.S., but Says He Backs Cole Memo*. NEWSWEEK. January 15, 2019

full of cash. Industry reports project the state's legal cannabis market will grow 19% annually over the next five years. But as state taxes rise and federal barriers remain, experts say higher prices for legal pot could drive buyers back to the black market. In Harborside's blockbuster case, an October tax court ruling from Holmes' court slapped the company with $11 million in back taxes from 2007 to 2012."[159]

This illustrates how Donald Trump could shut down every dispensary in America, *without* the cooperation of local law enforcement, or spending millions on extra DEA agents. He simply could do what happened in this case. Federal drug laws allow the IRS to fine dispensaries for drug trafficking. This case might be a "dry run." This could be practice for an industry shutdown.

Trump and Barr both have been accused of investigating this cannabis business because of prejudice against the industry. From the New York Times, we read:

> "Where things stand Two Justice Department officials sat before a congressional committee yesterday and stated plainly that President Trump and his attorney general, William Barr, had interfered in criminal and antitrust cases to advance their own personal interests. Aaron Zelinsky, a prosecutor who worked on the Russia investigation, told the House Judiciary Committee that senior officials had interfered with the prosecution of Roger Stone, a Trump ally, to seek a lighter sentence. "Roger Stone was treated differently because of politics," Zelinsky said. And John Elias, a senior career official in the antitrust division, said Barr had improperly sought investigations into the marijuana industry and California's dealings with automakers. "Personal dislike of the industry is not a valid basis upon which to ground an antitrust investigation," Elias said, referring to the cannabis cases."[160]

This case reveals a personal dislike for the industry. Of course, this should be no surprise, since President Trump erroneously believes that cannabis "permanently lowers the IQ," and assembled an "anti-cannabis cabinet."

President Trump Opposes Access for Military Vets

Many vets have suffered greatly for their service to this country. They return home from battle with severe pain, PTSD, and other serious conditions. According to studies, Cannabis could be a treatment. From *Science Daily*, we

---

159 ***California pot dispensary fights IRS tax case as costs mount for industry***. SAN FRANCISCO CHRONICLE. December 8, 2019

160 ***Bombshell Testimony Against Trump and Barr By Giovanni Russonello***. NEW YORK TIMES. June 25, 2020

read:

> "People suffering from post-traumatic distress disorder report that cannabis reduces the severity of their symptoms by more than half, at least in the short term, according to a recent study led by Carrie Cuttler, a Washington State University assistant professor of psychology. Cuttler and her colleagues analyzed data of more than 400 people who tracked changes in their PTSD symptoms before and after cannabis use with Strainprint, an app developed to help users learn what types of medical cannabis work best for their symptoms. The group collectively used the app more than 11,000 times over a 31-month period. The study, recently published in Journal of Affective Disorders, shows cannabis reduced the severity of intrusions, returning thoughts of a traumatic event, by about 62%; flashbacks by 51%, irritability by 67%, and anxiety by 57%"[161]

Three times the President has turned his back on our vets, by refusing to support bills that would give vets access to medical cannabis. We read:

> "At a cannabis conference last week, I overheard someone say, "we still don't know where Trump is on legalization." This is a long-held belief in the cannabis industry. Leafly said as much about then-candidate Trump in 2016. But it's worn thin over the years. This week it officially became a delusion. Here's what happened. In Congress, the House Veterans' Affairs Committee held a hearing Tuesday on three bills that would reduce restrictions on veterans' access to medical cannabis. One bill would allow VA healthcare providers to write state-legal medical cannabis recommendations for veterans who qualify. (Federal law currently prohibits them from doing so.) A separate bill would direct the VA to conduct a clinical study on the risks and benefits of medical marijuana. A third would prevent the VA from stripping veterans of their hard-earned benefits just because they consume state-legal cannabis. The Trump administration opposed all three. That [is] not merely nonsensical. It's cruel."[162]

Because Cannabis gives relief from PTSD, President Trump's action indirectly put the lives of our veterans at risk. They are a high risk for suicide. From Reuters, we read:

> "U.S. veterans with post-traumatic stress disorder (PTSD) are more likely than typical Americans to die of causes including suicide and accidental injuries, a recent study suggests. PTSD

---

161 *Cannabis temporarily relieves PTSD symptoms, study suggests.* SCIENCE DAILY. June 9, 2020
162 *Trump Opposes Cannabis Legalization* LEAFY. May 2, 2019

has previously been linked to increased risk for chronic health problems like heart disease, diabetes and immune disorders as well as a greater risk of premature death, researchers note in the American Journal of Preventive Medicine. But studies to date haven't offered a clear picture of what causes might be driving higher mortality rates among veterans with PTSD." [163]

President Trump does not understand their dilemma. He never suffered from PTSD. He never went to war. But in order to put the brakes on cannabis reforms, he denies them access to this medicine. He would rather further his agenda, than help these vets. With PTSD, vets are also at a greater risk for opiate addiction, which leads to heroin. From American Addiction Centers, we read:

> "Very few veterans ever thought they would find themselves struggling with a heroin addiction, yet it's a troubling trend that's on the rise. According to Veterans of Foreign Wars (VFW), since 2002, the number of U.S. veterans suffering from opioid addiction has doubled. A variety of risk factors, including difficulty returning to civilian life, struggles with post-traumatic stress disorder (PTSD), and chronic pain all increase the likelihood that veterans will fall into a pattern of substance abuse. The following article will discuss these risk factors in detail and provide advice for how loved ones can help a veteran struggling with addiction." (Heroin Addiction in Veterans. March 17, 2020[164])

Medical cannabis is safer than opiates. How can President Trump be so concerned with the "opiate crisis," yet support laws, and policies that deny cannabis to our vets? Veterans groups have asked for access to medical cannabis for years. We read:

> "One of the nation's most conservative veterans' groups is appealing to President Donald Trump to reclassify marijuana to allow large-scale research into whether cannabis can help troops suffering from post-traumatic stress disorder. The change sought by The American Legion would conflict with the strongly anti-marijuana positions of some administration leaders, most vocally Attorney General Jeff Sessions. Under current rules, doctors with the Department of Veterans Affairs cannot even discuss marijuana as an option with patients. But the alternative treatment is gaining support in the medical community, where some researchers hope pot might prove more effective than traditional pharmaceuticals in controlling PTSD symptoms and reducing the record number of veteran suicides. "We are not

163 **Vets with PTSD at increased risk of death from suicide, accidents**. REUTERS. June 26, 2019
164 **Heroin Addiction in Veterans**. March 17, 2020 AMERICAN ADDICTION CENTERS.

asking for it to be legalized," said Louis Celli, the national director of veterans affairs and rehabilitation for the American Legion, which with 2.4 million members is the largest U.S. veterans' organization. "There is overwhelming evidence that it has been beneficial for some vets. The difference is that it is not founded in federal research because it has been illegal."[165]

Vets are faced with a horrible choice because of this Administration. Either they struggle with PTSD symptoms, possibly killing themselves in the process, use more dangerous prescription drugs to deal with their symptoms, or break the law. Some of the most decorated vets have killed themselves due to combat depression, and PTSD. Because of federal laws, many vets go to the black market for their cannabis—out of fear:

> "According to the Marijuana Policy Project just under 2 million Californians, or around 3.4 percent of the state's population, get prescriptions for medical marijuana each year. But because of federal drug laws that still consider marijuana to be as dangerous as heroin, the Department of Veterans Affairs will not prescribe marijuana to its patients, even if they are totally disabled like Alex. "I use cannabis for PTSD [Post-Traumatic Stress Disorder], anxiety, hypervigilance," says Alex, who is being identified by a family name for privacy reasons. Alex is a Marine who deployed twice to Iraq from 2004 to 2007. He fought in the Second Battle of Fallujah, one of the fiercest battles in the Iraq War."[166]

Forcing vets to the black market for cannabis puts their lives at even greater risk, from criminals, and the police. Furthermore, if a vet gets caught with cannabis, they can lose their housing:

> "On that foggy February morning, her case would be presented to three judges at the University of Pittsburgh School of Law. And unless those judges side with her, she will be forced to choose between medical marijuana, which is legal in Pennsylvania but not under federal law, and federal public housing assistance. "I never thought that taking my medicine could lead to homelessness," Mary, 68, said. "But here we are."[167]

Homelessness among veterans is a big problem. The U.S. Department of Housing and Urban Development estimates that "...about 40,000 vets are

---

165 _ibid_

166 ***How Federal Marijuana Policy Is Pushing Veterans into the Black Market.*** POLITICO. March 27, 2020

167 NATIONAL COALITION FOR HOMELESS VETERANS

homeless on any given night.[168]" Vets are being denied housing because they want to treat their conditions with a safer substance. Cannabis is safer than tranquilizers, opiates, alcohol, and numerous legal prescriptions.

40,000 people are in prison for cannabis related offenses[169]. The policy of Donald Trump forces vets to risk this incarceration, in order to treat an illness they got for serving their country. One vet was sentenced to 5 years in prison:

> "West Alabama District Attorney Andy Hamlin defended the court decision to revoke Sean Worsley's probation, sending the Black disabled veteran to state prison for 60 months on felony marijuana charges. Hamlin spoke to APR in a phone interview about the case. Sean Worsley is a Black disabled veteran who was arrested on felony marijuana charges in Gordo in Pickens County in August 2016. Advocates for marijuana legalization, sentencing reform and for veterans have denounced Worsley's treatment by the Alabama court system. On April 28 a circuit judge in Alabama revoked the Arizona man's Alabama probation, so he faces spending 60 months of his life as a guest of the Alabama Department of Corrections."[170]

President Trump supports federal laws that have allowed this abomination to happen. No vet should go to jail for treating themselves with a plant that is safer than many prescription drugs. No vet should lose their housing, or be forced to choose between suicide, and obeying federal laws. President Trump's words "I support medical 100 percent" are hollow, and a lie to every veteran who believed he would support cannabis reforms.

---

168 *ibid*

169 **40K People Are In Prison For Cannabis In The US: Here's How Steve DeAngelo, Damian Marley And Stephen Marley Are Helping Them**. By Javier Hasse. FORBES. September 26, 2019

170 **DA defends imprisonment of disabled vet for marijuana charges**. ALABAMA POLITICAL REPORTER. June 17, 2020

CHAPTER 8:
THE WAR BETWEEN CANNABIS AND OPIUM

Big Money has corrupted politics. This problem is not confined to the United States Congress, or Presidents, but extends to the four corners of the earth, and throughout history. Today, pharmaceutical companies are one of the largest contributers to political campaigns. Politicians take this money, and refuse to legalize cannabis. Little has changed. Cannabis is in direct competition with opium, because both drugs alleviate pain.

Cannabis can be grown by anyone, in various climates. The opium poppy grows in specific locations, and must be refined. This makes it more valuable to drug companies. If cannabis becomes legal, anyone can grow it free, to use as a medicine. Opiates are more valuable because pharmaceutical companies have more control over it's sale and production.

Studies have been conducted that reveal which industries are against cannabis legalization. These are the five largest contributors:

1. Police Unions. Police get federal money to continue the drug war.
2. Private Prisons. Receive money for those incarcerated.
3. Alcohol Companies.
4. Pharmaceutical Companies
5. Prison Guard Unions[171]

---

171 ***The Top Five Special Interest Groups Lobbying To Keep Marijuana Illegal*** By Lee Fang. REPUBLIC REPORT.

The Two Biggest Industries against Cannabis: Alcohol and the Pharmaceutical Industry

The top two donors against the cannabis are the alcohol, and pharmaceutical companies. They give the most money to politicians, ad campaigns, and anti-cannabis groups. Because cannabis is in direct competition with alcohol, the booze industry contributes large sums of money against legalization. In the *Intercept*, we read:

> "...legalized pot is being heavily bankrolled by alcohol and pharmaceutical companies, terrified that they might lose market share. On the heels of a filing last week that revealed that a synthetic cannabis company is financing the opposition to legal marijuana in Arizona comes a new disclosure this week that a beer industry group made one of the largest donations to an organization set up to defeat legalization in Massachusetts. The Beer Distributors PAC, an affiliate that represents 16 beer-distribution companies in Massachusetts, gave $25,000 to the Campaign for a Safe and Healthy Massachusetts, tying it for third place among the largest contributors to the anti-pot organization."[172]

The alcohol industry gave $25,000 to "the Campaign for a Safe and Healthy Massachusetts." This is hypocritical, and laughable. Alcohol is far worse than cannabis, killing thousands each year by overdose—called "alcohol poisoning." Joining with the alcohol industry against cannabis, is the pharmaceutical industry:

> "Indeed, alcohol and pharma groups have been quietly backing antimarijuana efforts across the country. Besides Insys, the Arizona Wine and Spirits Wholesale Association gave one of the largest donations to the state's anti-legalization campaign when it paid $10,000 to Arizonans for Responsible Drug Policy. And the Beer Distributors PAC recently donated $25,000 to the Campaign for a Safe and Healthy Massachusetts, making it the state's third-largest backer of the opposition to recreational cannabis. Purdue Pharma and Abbott Laboratories, makers of the painkiller OxyContin and Vicodin, respectively, are among the largest contributors to the AntiDrug Coalition of America, according to a report in the Nation. And the Pharmaceutical Research and Manufacturers of America, considered one of marijuana's biggest opponents, spent nearly $19m on lobbying in 2015. The plant's threat to the alcohol industry is difficult to chart. Some researchers claim consumers

---

172 *Alcohol Industry Bankrolls fight against legal Pot in Battle of the Buzz.*
THE INTERCEPT. September 14, 2016

substitute alcohol with marijuana when the plant is legalized. But in Colorado, which legalized recreational marijuana in 2014, that scenario has not played out. Alcohol sales there have increased since cannabis legalization, according to state tax data...For big pharma, however, an expanding amount of data explains their fears. Opiate overdoses dropped by roughly 25% in states that have legalized medical marijuana compared to states that have prohibited sales of the plant, according to a 2014 study from the Journal of the American Medical Association. The study implies that people could be using medical marijuana to treat their pain rather than opioid painkillers, or they're taking lower doses. And research published this year by the University of Georgia shows that Medicare prescriptions for drugs used to treat chronic pain and anxiety dropped in states that have legalized medical marijuana. Medicare saved roughly $165m in 2013, according to the study, which estimated that expenditures for Medicare Part D, the portion of the government-funded health insurance program that subsidizes prescription drug costs, would drop by $470m annually if medical marijuana were legalized nationally."[173]

Already the legalization of cannabis has taken business from both of these companies. People are choosing not to have hangovers, and a safer, less toxic medication. The Pharmaceutical industry will loose billions of dollars, if cannabis is legalized. From *Civilized*, we read:

"$18.5 Billion Less For Big Pharma If All 50 States Legalize Medical Marijuana: Study. Nationwide medical marijuana legalization could take a multi-billion dollar bite out of the pharmaceutical industry, according to the latest research from analytics firm New Frontier Data. In a study titled 'From Prescription to Recommendation: How Cannabis Could Disrupt the Pharmaceutical Industry', researchers write that if medical cannabis were legalized in all 50 states, pharmaceutical expenditures on the top nine conditions commonly treated by medical cannabis could fall an estimated $18.5 billion between 2016 and 2019."[174]

18 Billion dollars is a lot of money to lose. However, the recent actions of President Trump could help offset this loss. Drug companies will be able to patent cannabinoid combinations under the new rules, while THC, and CBD remain on Schedule 1. Full implementation of these rules would take away your right to access this natural substance.

These companies have allies in Congress. In fact, some of the same

173 *Inside big pharma's fight to block recreational marijuana*. THE GUARDIAN. October 22, 2016
174 *$18.5 Billion Less For Big Pharma If All 50 States Legalize Medical Marijuana: Study*. CIVILIZED

companies that lobbied for a provision *easing* opiate restrictions, are against the legalization of cannabis. From *Forbes*, we read:

> "Senator Calls Out Big Pharma For Opposing Legal Marijuana. A prominent Democratic U.S. senator is slamming pharmaceutical companies for opposing marijuana legalization. "To them it's competition for chronic pain, and that's outrageous because we don't have the crisis in people who take marijuana for chronic pain having overdose issues," Sen. Kirsten Gillibrand of New York said. "It's not the same thing. It's not as highly addictive as opioids are."[175]

Companies who sell opiates are in direct competition with cannabis. For over one hundred and fifty years, money has financed this effort in several countries. This is the cannabis-opium "war." Pharmaceutical money has influenced every corner of our government, and the governments of foreign nations. Many President's, Congressmen, DEA, and FDA officials have received this money. The possibly of rewards, kickbacks, or future employment is endless.

Congress, and The FDA Influenced by Pharmaceutical Companies

The Food and Drug Administration has denied the medical properties of cannabis for years. One physician who chaired a committee at the FDA, spoke out against financial corruption at the agency. We read:

> "Dr. Raeford Brown, a pediatric anesthesia specialist at the UK Kentucky Children's Hospital and chair of the Food and Drug Administration (FDA) Committee on Analgesics and Anesthetics, has been openly critical of big pharma and the lack of proper oversight from the FDA. Despite many politicians, particularly declared presidential candidates, beginning to speak out against big pharma, Brown does not think that anything will come out of it "because Congress is owned by pharma." "The pharmaceutical industry pours millions of dollars into the legislative branch every single year," he told Yahoo Finance. " In 2016, they put $100 million into the elections. That's a ton of money."[176]

It has been discovered that numerous people who advise the FDA receive massive amounts of money, or rewards, from drug companies. From Science Magazine, we read:

> "In examining compensation records from drug companies to physicians who advised FDA on whether to approve 28 psychopharmacologic, arthritis, and cardiac or renal drugs

175 *Senator Calls Out Big Pharma For Opposing Legal Marijuana*. FORBES. February 23, 2018
176 *FDA medical adviser: 'Congress is owned by pharma'*. YAHOO NEWS. March 28, 2019

between 2008 and 2014, Science found widespread after-the-fact payments or research support to panel members. The agency's safeguards against potential conflicts of interest are not designed to prevent such future financial ties. Other apparent conflicts may have also slipped by: Science found that at the time of or in the year leading up to the advisory meetings, many of those panel members—including Halperin—received payments or other financial support from the drugmaker or key competitors for consulting, travel, lectures, or research. FDA did not publicly note those financial ties... Such money—including "associated research" funding that nearly always supports principal investigators—affects a scientist's career advancement, compensation, or professional influence."[177]

We cannot ignore the possible connections, although motive is hard to prove. Despite hard-core scientific evidence, the FDA continues to deny the medicinal properties of cannabis. At the same time, the pharmaceutical companies have given millions of dollars against the legalization of cannabis, and at the same time, advisors for the FDA have received direct payments from the same companies. All of these companies make drugs that are all in competition with cannabis. These are facts. You draw your own conclusions about collusion.

Here is a breakdown of all the money being given by drug companies to candidates, and committees:

"This observational study, which analyzed publicly available data on campaign contributions and lobbying in the US from 1999 to 2018, found that the pharmaceutical and health product industry spent $4.7 billion, an average of $233 million per year, on lobbying the US federal government; $414 million on contributions to presidential and congressional electoral candidates, national party committees, and outside spending groups; and $877 million on contributions to state candidates and committees. Contributions were targeted at senior legislators in Congress involved in drafting health care laws and state committees that opposed or supported key referenda on drug pricing and regulation."[178]

It appears to me, that if the drug companies did not spend so much money trying to bribe elected officials, people on advisory panels, or spend tons of money on advertisements— maybe they could charge a little less for prescription drugs. An average of $233 million a year in contributions by

177 *Hidden conflicts? Pharma payments to FDA advisers after drug approvals spark ethical concerns.* SCIENCE MAGAZINE. July 5, 2018
178 *Lobbying Expenditures and Campaign Contributions by the Pharmaceutical and Health Product Industry in the United States, 1999-2018* PUBMED. May, 2020

companies that are against their competitor—cannabis. And companies that *only* manufacture opiates have also given money to stop cannabis reforms:

> "AN EMBATTLED pharmaceutical company that sells the powerful painkiller fentanyl has donated $500,000 toward defeating a ballot initiative that would make recreational use of marijuana legal under Arizona law. It's hard to imagine a more sinister donor than Insys Therapeutics Inc. in the eyes of pot legalization proponents, who long have claimed drug companies want to keep cannabis illegal to corner the market for drugs, some addictive and dangerous, that relieve pain and other symptoms. Insys currently markets just one product, according to an August ling with the Securities and Exchange Commission: a sublingual fentanyl spray it calls Subsys. Two former company employees pleaded not guilty last month to federal charges related to an alleged kickback scheme to get doctors to prescribe Subsys."[179]

This is nothing new. As stated earlier, opium money has been used in various ways by governments, and corporations to oppose cannabis legalization, because it is a safer painkiller that can be grown freely in many environments. That makes it a serious competitor.

Unethical Collaboration

Several studies performed at Harvard, and various Universities across the country, have repeated the same charges about cannabis, year after year—*schizophrenia, heart attacks, strokes, etc*. At the same time, many of the same scientists have ties to pharmaceutical companies. One speaker at Harvard questioned the ethics of this collaboration:

> 'In describing the evolution of the relationship between the academy and industry, Angell focused on two specific domains. The first was that of clinical research. Because the FDA requires for approval that pharmaceutical companies demonstrate the safety and effectiveness (as compared to a placebo) of their products through trials involving live human subjects, and because those companies lack ready access to live human subjects, it has, for many years, been standard practice within the pharmaceutical industry to outsource these trials to academic medical centers. As recently as the mid-1980s, Angell recounted, this outsourcing took the form of companies giving money to medical centers to test their products and hoping for the best. In other words, companies took no role in designing or analyzing the trials involving their

---

179 *Fentanyl Maker Donates Big to Campaign Opposing Pot Legalization Pro-legalization campaign says 'we are truly shocked.'* US NEWS. Sept. 8, 2016

products, or in authoring and publishing the results. Clinical research funding was, as Angell put it, "at arm's length." As time went on, however, and as the pharmaceutical industry's financial clout increased, "arm's length" funding was steadily replaced by a much more hands-on counterpart, as it has now become entirely standard for pharmaceutical companies to have a direct hand in both the design and analysis of clinical trials, and in the authorship and (non)publication of results. Academic physicians are often, as Angell puts it, reduced to the role of "hired hands," carrying out trials as they are told and signing their names to ghost-authored reports. In addition to this shift in the character of clinical trials, Angell continued, direct financial ties between industry and both individual academic physicians and academic medical centers as wholes have become ever more pervasive. In a recent poll, Angell observed, a staggering 94% of surveyed physicians acknowledged receiving financial compensation of some form from pharmaceutical companies, ranging from small perks such as free gifts and meals to stipendiary speaking invitations and salaried positions as industry consultants. Academic medical centers, for their part, have been hesitant to clamp down on these apparent conflicts of interest insofar as they too have developed such direct financial ties, both in the form of a dependence on industry for research funding and in the form of potential compensation by industry for in-house discoveries."[180]

Medical colleges receive donations from drug companies, and it is hard to guess how much this effects the curriculum, and studies performed. Some studies are designed to be anti-cannabis, and repeated throughout the news. Fortunately, the average person does not keep up with the news, and if they haven't witnessed cannabis causing these problems *in real life*, are likely to ignore these reports.

Conflicts of Interest in a "Cannabis-Heart Attack" Study

In a previous chapter, we examined the claim that cannabis causes strokes or heart attacks. These studies, recycled year, after year, appear suspicious only because of their repetition, and their flawed method of "self-reporting" cannabis use. Cannabis use "sometime in a month" cannot be linked to any of these problems.

Some scientists who performed these studies might have conflicts of interest. Of course, it is impossible to know for certain if a scientist will receive money from a pharmaceutical company five, or ten years later. Some of these researchers have had strong ties with international pharmaceutical firms. For instance, in the study ***Marijuana Use in Patients With Cardiovascular Disease:***

180 ***Drug Companies and Medicine: What Money Can Buy***. HARVARD (thesis). December 10, 2009

JACC Review Topic of the Week, two of the researchers had multiple ties to the pharmaceutical industry. They worked for companies that produced drugs in direct competition with cannabis. One researcher, Dr Blankstein, received research support from the companies *Amgen and Astellas.*

Amgen Inc –a biopharmaceutical company. They manufacture a drug in direct competition with cannabis:

Etanercept, *sold under the brand name Enbrel among others, is a biopharmaceutical that treats autoimmune diseases by interfering with tumor necrosis factor (TNF, a soluble inflammatory cytokine) by acting as a TNF inhibitor.*
• THC treats autoimmune diseases[181], interferes with tumor necrosis factor TNF[182]

This researcher also had ties to Astelles, a Multinatinal Japanese pharmaceutical company. This company makes many drugs in competition with cannabis:

Advagraf, Prograf and Astagraf XL -Organ rejection
    THC prevents organ rejection[183]
AmBisome, Mycamine and Cresemba-Antifungal
    THC is anti-fungal[184]
Amevive-psoriasis
    THC treats psoriasis[185]

---

181 ***Marijuana shows potential in treating autoimmune disease*** June 2, 2014 SCIENCE DAILY. University of South Carolina "Summary: Researchers have discovered a novel pathway through which marijuana's main active constituent, THC, can suppress the body's immune functions. The recent findings show that THC can change critical molecules of epigenome called histones, leading to suppression of inflammation."
182 ***Cannabinoids, Endocannabinoids and Cancer***. June 3, 2012. CANCER METASTASIS REVIEWS. PUBMED. June 3, 2012.
183 ***Do Cannabinoids have a therapeutic role in transplantation?*** "Cannabinoids have emerged as powerful drug candidates for the treatment of inflammatory and autoimmune diseases due to their immunosuppressive properties. While significant clinical and experimental data on the use of cannabinoids as anti-inflammatory agents exist in many autoimmune disease settings, virtually no studies have been performed on their potential role in transplant rejection. Here we suggest a theoretical role for the use of cannabinoids in preventing allograft rejection. While the psychotropic properties of CB1 agonists limit their clinical use, CB2 agonists may offer a new avenue to selectively target immune cells involved in allograft rejection. Moreover, development of mixed CB1/CB2 agonists that cannot cross the blood-brain barrier may help prevent their undesired psychotropic properties. In addition, manipulation of endocannabinoids in vivo by activating their biosynthesis and inhibiting cellular uptake and metabolism may offer yet another pathway to regulate immune response during allograft rejection."
184 ***Fungal biotransformation of cannabinoids: potential for new effective drugs*** https:// pubmed.ncbi.nlm.nih.gov/19333876/
185 ***Is Cannabis an Effective Treatment for Psoriasis? Susan York Morris***. HEALTHLINE. July 11,

Enfortumab vedotin, Xtandi ,Tarceva-anticancer

    THC is anticancer[186]

Lexiscan- Vasodialator

    THC is a vasodialator[187]

Protopic-Eczema

    THC can treat eczema[188]

Symoron (methadone HCL)-opioid treatment

    THC treats opioid addiction[189]

Vibativ-Antibiotic

    THC, CBD gram positive antibiotic[190]

Now, despite having ties these companies, it is hard to prove influence. But it is certainly possible, considering all the money these companies could lose. Another researcher had ties to *multiple* pharmaceutical companies:

> "Dr. Bhatt has served on the Advisory Board of Cardax, Cereno Scientific, PhaseBio, and Regado Biosciences...has served as Chair of the American Heart Association Quality Oversight Committee... AEGIS-II executive committee funded by CSL Behring)...Duke Clinical Research Institute...has received research funding from ...Amarin, Amgen, AstraZeneca, Bayer, Boehringer Ingelheim, Bristol-Myers Squibb, Chiesi, CSL Behring, Eisai, Ethicon, Forest Laboratories, Fractyl, Idorsia, Ironwood, Ischemix, Lilly...PhaseBio, PLx Pharma, Pfizer, Regeneron, Roche, Sanofi, Synaptic, and The Medicines Company..." [191]

A web has been weaved between our politicians, government agencies, medical schools, physicians with the pharmaceutical industry. This web also ties people together that oppose the legalization of cannabis. This web has weakened opiate laws, and possibly affected the Centers for Disease Control (CDC). This agency has also received money from the pharmaceutical industry. From *ASH Clinical News*, we read:

2019

186 *Anticancer mechanisms of cannabinoids*. CURRENT ONCOLOGY. PUBMED March 23, 2016

187 *Cardiovascular Pharmacology of Cannabinoids*. HANDBOOK OF EXPERIMENTAL PHARMACOLOGY. PUBMED. February 4, 2008.

188 *Marijuana may help cure eczema, according to researchers*. By Chelsea Ritschel. THE INDEPENDENT. June 4, 2018.

189 *Medical cannabis patterns of use and substitution for opioids & other pharmaceutical drugs, alcohol, tobacco, and illicit substances; results from a cross-sectional survey of authorized patients*. HARM REDUCTION JOURNAL. January 28, 2019.

190 *Study reveals antibiotic potential of cannabis compound* By Nikki Hancocks NUTRA. March 2, 2020

191 *Marijuana Use in Patients With Cardiovascular Disease: JACC Review Topic of the Week*. SCIENCE DIRECT. January, 2020

"During fiscal years 2014 through 2018, the CDC Foundation received $79.6 million from companies like Pfizer, Biogen, and Merck. Since it was created by Congress in 1995, the nonprofit organization has accepted $161 million from corporations. Public Citizen, Knowledge Ecology International, Liberty Coalition, Project on Government Oversight, and U.S. Right to Know filed the petition. The groups are concerned about the pharmaceutical industry's possible undue influence on medical research and practice."[192]

The CDC appears to be part of this opiate "web." Remember, data was falsified in the *National Health Interview Survey*. Since they received this money, are other interviews flawed? We just don't know. Many believed news reports have been based on these studies, and at least one of them was based on inaccurate data.

Since the end of World War 2, money from drug companies have corrupted almost every aspect of medical science in the United States. The same people who are bought off, are also against cannabis. They fail to grasp how cannabis could really help many sick people, so they believe lies possibly fed to them by corporate allies.

The Beginning of the Cannabis-Opium "War"

The modern war between cannabis and opium began about one hundred and seventy five years ago. The weapons of this war back then were the same as today—*disinformation, and money*. The British government traded with China, purchasing tea with silver. At that time opium was also outlawed, because the British government realized how addictive, and dangerous it was. Yet over time, they decided to pay for their tea *a different way*.

So in 1858, the British government legalized the opium trade. They harvested, and processed opium in India, and traded, or sold it to the Chinese as a pain killer. However, there was a safer, less addictive drug used throughout India at that time—Cannabis.

Prior to the legalization of opium, a physician W. B. O'Shaughnessy, published "**On the preparations of the Indian hemp, or gunjah (Cannabis Indica), their effects on the animal system in health, and their utility in the treatment of tetanus 6 and other convulsive disorders**" in 1839. This paper recorded many medicinal properties of cannabis, including the treatment of seizures. That's right, *almost two centuries before recent news reports*, it was known that cannabis could treat epilepsy. This paper also revealed that cannabis could treat pain.

Because of the vast amounts of money to be made in the opium trade, the use of cannabis as a medicinal drug became a problem—especially in

192 *CDC Pressed to Acknowledge Industry Funding*. ASH CLINICAL NEWS. November 18, 2019

India, where the poppies were being harvested. The Indian population who harvested the poppies preferred cannabis over opium, both as a pain killer and an intoxicant. This was a bad advertisement. So, what happened? People in the British Government made these false charges against cannabis:

- It caused insanity
- It caused violence
- It caused physical harm
- It caused immorality

After years of these accusations, and threats of prohibition, a commission was assembled to study this issue. It investigated over one thousand cannabis users:

> "The Commission actually met for the first time in Calcutta on 3 August 1893 (1:4). Between this date and 6 August of the following year, when the study was finished (1:361), the Commission received evidence from 1,193 witnesses (1:12). Field trips were made to thirty cities in eight provinces and Burma from the end of October 1893 through the latter part of April 1894 (1:9-10). Eighty-six meetings for examination of witnesses transpired during the inquiry. Actual participation of the members of the Commission was duly noted and reported - a custom that it might be worthwhile to revive."[193]

On the physical effects, the commission stated:

> "The Commission have now examined all the evidence before them regarding the effects attributed to hemp drugs. It will be well to summarize briefly the conclusions to which they come. It has been clearly established that the occasional use or hemp in moderate doses may be beneficial; but this use may be regarded as medicinal in character."

The commission concluded cannabis does not cause mental illness:

> 'In respect to the alleged mental effects of the drugs, the Commission have come to the conclusion that the moderate use of hemp drugs produces no injurious effects on the mind. It may indeed be accepted that in the case of specially marked neurotic diathesis, even the moderate use may produce mental injury. For the slightest mental stimulation or excitement may have that effect in such cases. But putting aside these quite exceptional cases, the moderate use of these drugs produces no mental

---

193 *The Hemp Drugs Commission*. WIKIPEDIA.

injury."

It was the conclusion of the committee:

"Viewing the subject generally, it may be added that the moderate use of these drugs is the rule, and that the excessive use is comparatively exceptional. The moderate use practically produces no ill effects. In all but the most exceptional cases, the injury from habitual moderate use is not appreciable. The excessive use may certainly be accepted as very injurious, though it must be admitted that in many excessive consumers the injury is not clearly marked. The injury done by the excessive use is, however, confined almost exclusively to the consumer himself; the effect on society is rarely appreciable. It has been the most striking feature in this inquiry to find how little the effects of hemp drugs have obtruded themselves on observation. The large number of witnesses of all classes who professed never to have seen these effects, the vague statements made by many who professed to have observed them, the very few witnesses who could so recall a case as to give any definite account of it, and the manner in which a large proportion of these cases broke down on the first attempt to examine them, are facts which combine to show most clearly how little injury society has hitherto sustained from hemp drugs."

This commission studied a large group of cannabis users, and denied all of these charges against the drug. But these lies were told for a purpose. It wasn't because they really cared about the Indian population, proven by the harsh working conditions. No, a competing industry was *losing money*, so a government *pretended* it cared.

Now, let's move ahead over 150 years. Richard Nixon began the drug war, which was another battle in the war against cannabis. In 1970, the Controlled Substance Act was passed. The Shaffer Commission was assembled by Congress to investigate these charges against marijuana:

- It caused insanity
- It caused violence
- It caused physical harm
- It caused immorality

As the committee that studied cannabis use in India about one hundred years previously, the Shaffer commission studied cannabis users, and found *no evidence* that cannabis caused any of these problems, and recommended it be decriminalized.

Their recommendation was rejected by President Nixon, and he ordered it to be placed on Schedule 1, where it remains today. Now, history is repeating itself. President Trump has assembled a special cabinet to combat the legalization of cannabis by claiming it causes *violence, insanity, physical harm, and immorality.*

President Trump Doesn't Receive Any Opiate Donations?

In a "confidence game," an initial investment is made to convince the "mark" of your sincerity. Con artists are not the only people who use this method—it is also used in business. President Trump has performed some actions that appear admirable, but could be an attempt to deceive. For instance, he has donated his fourth quarter salary of $100,000 toward fighting opiate addiction. However, he is worth about *two billion dollars*, so this minuscule amount is nothing, compared to his net worth.

Sometimes public actions deflect from the actual truth. Earlier in 2019, President Trump announced that he would not take any money from companies that manufactured opiates:

> "President Donald Trump spurned campaign contributions from the pharmaceutical industry on Wednesday, calling the industry out for its role in a national opioid addiction epidemic. "I don't want their money," Trump said at an event on drug addiction in Atlanta. "They have got to do what is right."[194]

Since opiate addiction is taking many lives, it appears the President really cares. Unless this action is a ruse. He spoke these words last year. Yet, now we learn:

> "Donald Trump has benefited from more than $4.5 million in campaign funds linked to the deadly opioid epidemic ravaging the nation. The Trump campaign and the Republican National Committee raised the funds from heirs to the Johnson & Johnson fortune as well as Stewart Rahr, former head of Kinray, a pharmaceutical distributor. According to financial contributions flagged by American Bridge, a progressive opposition research organization, the Johnson family and Rahr donated $4,508,100 to Trump campaign efforts between late 2016 and February 2020. Woody Johnson, a Johnson & Johnson heir, owns more than $200 million worth of stock in the company. Over the past several years, he donated $2.17 million to help Trump's campaign, including $1 million for Trump's inaugural committee. In 2017, Trump nominated — and the Republican-led Senate subsequently approved —Johnson to be the U.S. ambassador to the United

---

194 ***Trump Says He Doesn't Want Campaign Donations From Pharma***
By Justin Sink and Bill Allison April 24, 2019

Kingdom."[195]

One contributor to the President's campaign is the heir to the Johnson and Johnson fortune, and Trump appointed him to be Ambassador to the United Kingdom. From this man, and many other pharmaceutical companies, Trump received $4, 500,000 in donations for his reelection. But he promised not to receive *any* money from the opiate industry, remember? His actions do not always match his words. These companies profit from selling several products—including opiates.

Opiate Influence, or Coincidence?

The President has received money from drug companies, as the FDA, medical schools, and almost every member of congress. But his actions have openly displayed obvious corporate cronyism. People from the same companies that contributed to the opioid epidemic have been nominated, and appointed in several cabinet level positions.

The President's connections add to this "pharmaceutical web." It is not beyond the imagination to believe these people have an influence on many decisions. Four companies were implicated in the opiate epidemic, and settled out of court before the trial began. President Trump has held stock, and appointed former CEO's from three of these companies. From CNN, we read:

> "Hours before the first federal trial in the opioid epidemic was set to begin, four pharmaceutical companies reached a settlement totaling $260 million. The four companies -- McKesson Corp., Cardinal Health Inc., AmerisourceBergen Corp. and Teva Pharmaceutical Industries Ltd. -- reached a settlement Monday morning with the two plaintiffs, Summit and Cuyahoga counties in Ohio. McKesson Corp., Cardinal Health Inc. and AmerisourceBergen Corp. will pay out a combined $215 million immediately, and Teva Pharmaceutical will pay $20 million, officials said at a press conference Monday. Teva will also be donating $25 million worth of Suboxone, according a source familiar with the settlement." (4 pharmaceutical companies accused in the opioid epidemic reach a $260 million settlement just before trial."[196]

The first company listed in this article is *McKensson Corporation.* In President Trump's effort to "jump-start" the economy, called *"the Great American Economic Revival Industry Groups,"* the CEO of McKesson Corporation, Brian Tyler is listed as an advisor, as well as Mike Kaufmann of Cardinal

---

195 ***Trump campaign is taking lots of cash from companies profiting off opioid epidemic*** By Dan Desai Martin AMERICAN INDEPENDENT March 4, 2020

196 ***4 pharmaceutical companies accused in the opioid epidemic reach a $260 million settlement just before trial.*** By Aaron Cooper, Kristina Sgueglia and Holly Yan. CNN. October 21, 2019

Health[197]. Both of these companies also were all part of the initial effort to coordinate the pandemic:

> "Maloney released a 13-page report ahead of Thursday's hearing that details committee's discussions to date with in-house legal counsel, senior officials procurement experts and other representatives from six leading distributors of medical equipment: Cardinal Health, Concordance Healthcare Solutions, Henry Schein, McKesson, Medline, and Owens & Minor. They labeled Trump's coordination not just inadequate but in many cases nonexistent in the pandemic's early months."[198]

According to this report, President Trump had *little* input in this coordination. If this report is true, pharmaceutical executives were basically running the show. But a Senate investigation has been launched, because their companies failed to provide the promised quantity of masks:

> "Three U.S. senators today demanded an investigation into Project Air Bridge, a Trump administration supply chain management project to import personal protective equipment (PPE) and other medical supplies during the COVID-19 pandemic. Dubbing the project "opaque," U.S. Senators Elizabeth Warren (D-Mass.), Chuck Schumer (D-N.Y.) and Richard Blumenthal (D-Conn.) also released new documents and information from the six major medical wholesalers or distribution companies involved in the project —Cardinal Health (NYSE:CAH), McKesson, Medline Industries, Henry Schein (NSDQ:HSIC), Owens & Minor (NYSE:OMI) and Concordance Healthcare Solutions. Warren and Blumenthal began investigating Project Air Bridge in April after multiple reports of seizures of supplies by federal officials and what they characterized in a news release as "political favoritism, cronyism, and price-gouging via third-party sellers." The companies' responses to the senators' requests for information left some questions unanswered, prompting the request for an investigation by the Congressional Pandemic Response Accountability Committee (PRAC). The companies' responses to the senators' initial inquiry are attached to the release."[199]

Another company implicated in the opiate epidemic was *Teva*

---

197 *President Trump taps North Texas businesses for economic revival task force*. By Taylor Tompkins DALLAS BUSINESS JOURNAL Apr 16, 2020
198 *Trump Appointees Held to House's Fire on Worsening US Pandemic*. By Brandi Bachman. COURTHOUSE NEWS SERVICE. July 2, 2020
199 *U.S. senators demand investigation of Trump COVID-19 supply chain effort*. By Nancy Crotti. MASSDEVICE. June 9, 2020

Pharmaceuticals. Teva also has close ties to this Administration, and it is possible criminal charges against them have been delayed due to political influence:

> "Today, Patients Over Pharma sent a letter to Attorney General William Barr calling on him to release details about the status of the Department of Justice's (DOJ) investigation into Teva Pharmaceuticals. Specifically, the letter seeks information regarding whether the long-running investigation has been influenced by Teva's lobbying, close ties to the Administration, or donations of hydroxychloroquine immediately following President Trump's endorsement of the anti-malarial drug as a COVID-19 treatment. This letter follows reporting that Teva "all but walked away" from settlement talks with the DOJ "essentially daring the Trump administration to file charges" against a company that appeared to be supporting President Trump's COVID-19 response efforts, as well as reporting that the DOJ had a May 31st deadline to decide whether to bring charges against Teva, drop the charges, or reach an agreement with the company to extend the statute of limitations –which passed without any information released on the status of the investigation."[200]

Three of the largest opiate manufacturers—implicated in the opiate epidemic—have ties to this Administration. President Trump has gone much further than being influenced by pharmaceutical money. He has appointed former CEO's to key positions in our government. For this reason alone, any action the President takes against cannabis should be suspect.

President Trump promised to bring down drug prices. He did sign an executive order to drop insulin prices[201], to the objections of these companies. But they were being sued for inflating the price *anyway*[202], and we have no idea what arrangement they might have after the election. Dropping the price of insulin works well for his reelection prospects, which these companies likely support.

Other connections are also on public display. President Trump appointed a lobbyist for McKesson to head the FDA:

> "Unfortunately, the answer is clear: Big Pharma has taken just a portion of its record profits and invested in doing everything possible to prevent any policy changes that would put its carve-outs, giveaways, sweetheart deals, or profits at risk. And

200 *Watchdog Group to Justice Department: Is Teva Pharmaceuticals Investigation Being Influenced By Political Pressure.* Press Release. ACCOUNTABLE. June 17, 2020
201 *Executive Order.* WHITEHOUSE.GOV https://www.whitehouse.gov/presidential-actions/ executive-order-access-affordable-life-saving-medications/
202 *Judge Dismisses RICO Claims, But 3 Insulin Makers Must Still Face Drug Pricing Lawsuit* By Kelly Davio. AJMC CENTER FOR BIOSIMILARS February 19, 2019

nowhere is this corruption more egregious than within Trump's administration. Here are just a few examples. It starts at the top. Before Azar joined the administration, he was a top executive getting paid millions of dollars by Eli Lilly, including a severance package of $1.6 million, which was paid out prior to joining the administration. Keagan Resler Lenihan — the chief of staff at the FDA and former senior counselor to the HHS secretary — ran lobbying efforts for the pharmaceutical company McKesson as senior director of government affairs from 2011-2016. In November, federal prosecutors launched a new criminal investigation into McKesson's opioid work; the company is currently facing an investor lawsuit regarding drug price-fixing. The director of the Domestic Policy Council for the White House is Joe Grogan. From 2011 to 2017, he was a lobbyist for the pharmaceutical company Gilead Sciences. The House Oversight Committee looked into Grogan's conflict of interest; Rep. Elijah Cummings said it appeared to "run afoul of the Trump Administration's own ethics rules." Since joining the administration, Grogan has worked to roll back drug pricing control efforts, including inviting a member of his former employer's advisory board to speak to a working group, ostensibly trying to bring down drug prices. The Atlantic reported that he "seems poised to take his momentum into drug pricing, pushing largely to maintain the 'status quo.'"[203]

Although part of an opinion piece, this quote accurately encapsulates all of Trump's connections. The President also sold stock in these companies as soon as he took office:

- McKesson: $100,000-$250,000.
- Johnson & Johnson: $100,000-$250,000.
- Gilead Sciences: $100,000-$250,000.
- Celgene: $100,000-$250,000[204].

There is connection between the stocks Trump once held, and the people he has appointed to key positions of power. He held stocks in *Gilead Sciences*. This company supplies the drug President Trump promotes to treat the coronavirus. They reaped huge profits, thanks to this Administration:

"Former presidential candidates Sens. Elizabeth Warren and Bernie Sanders slammed the Trump administration Thursday for giving Gilead Sciences a "windfall" deal to secure most of the

203 *Opinion: Trump Said He'd Battle Big Pharma. Instead, He Let It Run The White House* By Kyle Herrig BUZZFEED NEWS. January 24, 2020
204 *How Becoming President Cost Trump $3.75 Million*. By Sean Williams. MOTLEY FOOL. September 16, 2019

pharmaceutical company's supply of its coronavirus-fighting drug remdesivir with the United States. In a new letter addressed to U.S. Health and Human Services Secretary Alex Azar that was obtained by CNBC, Warren, Sanders and other lawmakers said the deal will give Gilead up to $500 million in revenue borne almost entirely by American taxpayers, "in whole or in part" through higher insurance premiums. "Outside analysts have concluded that 'The deal is amazingly good for Gilead's executives and shareholders and amazingly bad for everyone else—bad for taxpayers, terrible for public health, and unethical,'" the lawmakers wrote in the later dated Thursday."[205]

A former lobbyist for Giliad Sciences was director of the White House Domestic Policy Council:

"Joe Grogan, head of the White House Domestic Policy Council, intends to leave his position at the end of May... Grogan has served as the director of the White House Domestic Policy Council since February 2019, overseeing a broad array of policy issues including health care and regulation. Before that, he worked as a top health care official in the Office of Management and Budget beginning in 2017 and was a close ally of Mick Mulvaney, Trump's third chief of staff, whom Meadows replaced in March. Grogan worked as a lobbyist for drug company Gilead Sciences before joining the Trump administration."

The President appointed a lobbyist from this pharmaceutical company to oversee health care, and regulation. This is akin to putting a fox incharge of the henhouse. The President also held stock in the biopharmaceutical company *Celgene*. The Executive Chairman of this company worked on President Trump's transition team:

"BioCentury picked up a juicy bit of biotech-related presidential campaign news. Quoting sources, BioCentury says that Celgene EVP of corporate affairs Rich Bagger has taken a leave to work on Donald Trump's transition team. That won't get any flak from the top team at Celgene, as Executive Chairman Bob Hugin is a committed Republican and delegate pledged to back Trump at the Republican Convention this week."[206]

Trump considered the same man to head the Department of Health and Human Services (HHS):

205 *Sens. Elizabeth Warren and Bernie Sanders slam Trump for giving Gilead 'windfall' deal for coronavirus drug*. By Berkeley Lovelace Jr. CNBC. July 17, 2020
206 *Celgene EVP Bagger gets a plum assignment on Trump team.* By John Carrol. ENDPOINT NEWS. July 19, 2016

"Additionally, Celgene maintains a stash of cash overseas. Celgene, along with many other pharma companies, keeps a chunk of money it makes in overseas markets offshore to avoid paying high corporate tax rates it would be charged by bringing that money back. Citing a Bloomberg report Stat said the company has almost $7 billion in overseas banks. In addition to Hugin, Trump is also close to another Celgene executive, Rich Bagger. Celgene's executive vice president of corporate affairs and market access, Bagger took a leave of absence to helm the transition team of Donald Trump's presidential campaign. Bagger had been rumored to be on the short list as a potential Secretary of the Department of Health and Human Services, a role that ultimately went to Tom Price, who resigned in September. However, in November 2016, BioSpace reported that Bagger was returning to his role at Celgene."[207]

The President has nominated multiple people from the pharmaceutical industry into key positions of power. He has taken advice from them, appointed them to his transition team, had them basically coordinate the pandemic, and has given them opportunities to receive huge profits. Who knows what investments are shielded in tax shelters overseas? President Trump is in the position to reap great rewards from the same companies that have given millions against the legal cannabis industry.

Cabinet Positions

Numerous cabinet positions in the Trump Administration have been filled by people with ties to drug companies. These people are in positions to make decisions about cannabis, a competitor to many pharmaceutical drugs. Tom Price held investments in McKesson, before introducing a bill that would have increased company profits:

"Rep. Tom Price of Georgia, President Donald Trump's nominee for secretary of health and human services, invested up to $15,000 in a health company before introducing a bill that benefitted it, according to a report from USA Today. USA Today's Jayne O'Donnell reports that Price's investment broker bought $15,000 worth of McKesson stock in March and informed Price of the purchase in April. On May 12, Price introduced the Patient Access to Durable Medical Equipment Act, which in part stopped cuts of Medicare reimbursement for medical beds. McKesson, which produces medical beds, told investors that cuts in Medicare payments would be detrimental to its business

207 *The Complicated Relationship Between Celgene and President Trump.* By Alex Keown. BIOSPACE. Oct 30, 2017

in its annual report, filed a week before the bill was introduced, according to the report. The bill did not pass, but parts of it made their way into the recently passed 21st Century Cures Act, which Price, an orthopedic surgeon, did not support. Representatives from the Trump administration and HHS told USA Today that the McKesson investment didn't influence Price's legislation and that he had worked on multiple similar bills in the years before the investment as well."[208]

President Trump nominated Price, who coincidentally also held stocks in the same companies represented in key cabinet positions:

"The extent of potential conflicts for Price is unclear; they are the subject of ongoing investigations. According to reports from CNN last week, Price purchased between $1,000 and $15,000 in stock in leading medical-device company Zimmer Biomet in May 2016, just two weeks before introducing a law that would have delayed Medicare value-based purchasing rules that might decrease payments to companies like Zimmer Biomet. Later that year Zimmer Biomet's political action committee donated $1,000 to Price. Further reports indicate that Price also invested as much as $90,000 in 2016 in the pharmaceutical companies Eli Lilly, Bristol-Meyers Squibb, Amgen, McKesson, Biogen, and Pfizer, and co-sponsored a bill that these companies lobbied for that would have blocked a proposed change in Medicare reimbursement rates that would have specifically impacted them. None of these purchases came via mutual funds, which means his broker decided—at Price's general direction—to purchase these specific stocks based on information she had about their financial futures."[209]

After Tom Price resigned (because of $400,000 in travel bills for chartered flights[210],) the President nominated Alex Azar, who *also* has ties to the pharmaceutical industry:

"American Oversight today sued the Department of Health and Human Services to compel the release of communications between Secretary Alex Azar and the pharmaceutical industry —including Eli Lilly, where Azar worked until 2017. The administration has failed to provide final responses to several Freedom of Information Act requests, filed by American Oversight

208 *Trump's nominee for the top US healthcare job made a 4th shady investment in a health company.* By Bob Bryan. BUSINESS INSIDER. February 2, 2017

209 *Why Do Tom Price's Potential Conflicts of Interest Matter?* By Vann R. Newkirk II. THE ATLANTIC. January 19, 2017

210 *Tom Price resigns as health secretary over private flights and Trump criticism.* By Lauren Gambino. THE GUARDIAN. September 18, 2017.

in March, that sought records reflecting whether Azar or his staff having communicated with pharmaceutical industry groups and companies like Pfizer, AstraZeneca and Johnson & Johnson." (*Investigating HHS Secretary Alex Azar's Connections to Pharmaceutical Companies*. AMERICAN OVERSIGHT. August 27, 2019[211])

Not one, but *two* people the President nominated to head the Department of Health and Human Services had ties to the pharmaceutical industry. As stated before, these companies produce drugs in direct competition with cannabis. The President's nominee to head the Food and Drug Administration (FDA) also had past ties to these companies:

"NEWLY-RELEASED FINANCIAL disclosure documents show that Dr. Scott Gottlieb, President Trump's nominee to lead the Food and Drug Administration, has received significant payments from the opioid industry — while attacking attempts to deter the explosion of opioid pill mills. The FDA has some of the most significant authority in the federal government to oversee manufacturers of prescription painkillers. Gottlieb is set to appear for his confirmation hearing before the Senate Health, Education, Labor, and Pensions Committee at 10 a.m. Tomorrow. Gottlieb's disclosure statements, required under federal law, show that since the beginning of 2016 he has received almost $45,000 in speaking fees from firms involved in the manufacture and distribution of opioids. "Our country is in desperate need of an FDA commissioner who will take on the opioid lobby, not one who has a track record of working for it," said Dr. Andrew Kolodny, the co-director of Opioid Policy Research at Brandeis University, reacting to this information. Mallinckrodt Pharmaceuticals, the maker of a highly addictive generic oxycodone pill, paid Gottlieb $22,500 for a speech in London last November shortly after the U.S. presidential election. Prosecutors have charged that the firm ignored red flags and supplied as many as 500 million suspicious orders in Florida for its oxycodone product between 2008 and 2012." [212]

Donald Trump has nominated people with connections to the pharmaceutical industries to head *two* agencies responsible for the regulation of Health, and drugs. Other cabinet posts also are filled with people from this industry—which "coincidentally" wants to keep cannabis illegal as Donald Trump.

211 *Investigating HHS Secretary Alex Azar's Connections to Pharmaceutical Companies*. AMERICAN OVERSIGHT. August 27, 2019
212 *Donald Trump's Pick to Oversee Big Pharma is Addicted to Opioid-Industry Cash*. By Lee Fang. THE INTERCEPT. April 4 2017

One nominee, a former congressman, helped pass a law that weakened the DEA's ability to cite opiate distributors, and physicians, for violating federal prescription laws. This helped cause the opiate epidemic:

> "During his time in Congress, Marino has developed a cozy relationship with the drug distributors that his office would help oversee—and which stand to lose from a federal crackdown on painkiller distribution. Pharmaceutical distributors, which disseminate drugs to pharmacies across the country, were among the top contributors to Marino's House campaigns. They lobbied extensively to support legislation, signed into law last year, that Marino co-sponsored making it more difficult for the Drug Enforcement Agency to shut down pharmacies it suspects are diverting pills. Today, Marino's former chief of staff is a vice president at the National Association of Chain Drug Stores. When Marino was nominated, "my jaw dropped," says Andrew Kolodny, who directs opioid policy research at Brandeis university and leads Physicians for Responsible Opioid Prescribing. "I knew he was the guy who had championed the bill that weakened the DEA at a time when we need them to be able to do their job more effectively. If he was someone who cared about the opioid crisis, he never would have pushed through that bill." [213]

President Trump constantly laments about the opiate epidemic, yet he nominates the Congressman that help write the bill that contributed to this problem. This man is well-known for his opposition to any cannabis reforms— even CBD, *and* the Hemp Bill:

> "President Donald Trump's pick to head the nation's war on drugs: a man who once said drug users belong in a "hospital-slash-prison."...Marino is a former federal prosecutor with a history of voting against drug policy reforms. That puts him in line with other Trump administration figures — particularly Attorney General Jeff Sessions — who have moved from the more public health–oriented approach to drugs advocated by President Barack Obama's administration in favor of cracking down on drugs more through the criminal justice system. Given that Marino and Sessions will guide the offices most connected to federal drug policy, this suggests Trump is really intent on escalating the war on drugs. Marino's voting record suggests he's to the right of many of his Republican colleagues on the war on drugs. After he assumed office in 2011, he voted against a bipartisan measure

---

213 ***Drug Companies Sure Are Cozy With Trump's Pick to Solve the Opioid Crisis***. By Julia Lurie. MOTHER JONES. October 13, 2017

(which ultimately passed) that blocked the US Department of Justice from cracking down on medical marijuana businesses in states where medicinal pot is legal. He voted against a bill that would've let Veterans Affairs doctors recommend medical marijuana to patients. He opposed loosening restrictions on hemp and CBD, both of which are nonpsychoactive but have promising, respectively, industrial and medical uses." [214]

The man Donald Trump picked to head the "war on drugs," opposed any legal reforms on cannabis, CBD and Hemp. He believes all drug users– which would include cannabis consumers–should be locked up. Is it merely coincidence this man has had a close relationship with the pharmaceutical industry, which is also against the legalization of cannabis?

Opposition to Cannabis Reforms and Opiate Money in the Senate

Senate majority leader Mitch McConnell has refused to allow any pro-cannabis Bills on the Senate floor for a vote. Reforms that would have passed were blocked by this one man. He has said flatly, that he will not support legalizing Cannabis:

> "Senate Majority Leader (R-Ky.) on Tuesday told reporters he has no plan to support the legalization of marijuana as he pushes an effort to legalize hemp. "I do not have any plans to endorse the legalization of marijuana," he said, adding that marijuana and hemp are "two entirely separate plants." The top Republican in March to legalize hemp, taking it off the federal list of controlled substances and allowing it to be sold as an agricultural product. Hemp has small amounts of THC, the main psychoactive component of marijuana. "It is a different plant. It has an illicit cousin which I choose not to embrace," McConnell said of hemp on Tuesday."[215]

McConnell's reluctance to the legalization of cannabis might be more than misguided fear of this plant. His actions could be shaded—by pharmaceutical donations:

> "Senate Majority Leader Mitch McConnell announced in September that he would block any consideration of a bill to lower prescription drug costs. By the end of December, he had raked in more than $50,000 in contributions from political

---

214 *Trump's new drug czar nominee once said drug users belong in a "hospital-slash-prison" Trump's pick signals a continued escalation of the war on drugs.* By German Lopez VOX. Sep 5, 2017

215 *McConnell: I won't support legalizing marijuana.* By Jacqueline Thomsen. THE HILL. May 8, 2018

action committees and individuals tied to the pharmaceutical industry...On Oct. 16, McConnell received a $2,500 check from Takeda Pharmaceuticals' political action committee, according to McConnell's reports to the Federal Election Commission. The same campaign finance filings show that a few weeks after that, multinational pharmaceutical company Novartis' PAC also sent $2,500 to McConnell. Then, a PAC for another pharma company, Emergent BioSolutions, kicked in $2,500. By the end of December, McConnell's campaign reported, he had received at least $30,000 more from the corporate political action committees of Bluebird Bio ($2,500), Boehringer Ingelheim ($5,000), Greenwich Biosciences ($2,500), Teva USA ($10,000), and UCB ($2,500). According to filings from his Bluegrass Committee leadership PAC, Merck & Co. also contributed $5,000 to support McConnell and Sanofi donated $2,500. Over that time period, McConnell's campaign also received $5,000 from Gilead Sciences CEO Daniel O'Day, $2,000 from Amgen lobbyist Helen Rhee, and $5,600 from his former policy director and current Pharmaceutical Research and Manufacturers of America registered lobbyist Hazen Marshall."[216]

Senator McConnell blocked a vote on a bill to lower drug costs after receiving more than $50,000 in contributions from companies that were against it. Similiarly, the Senator blocks any votes on cannabis reforms. He would not allow a vote on a bill to reform banking laws, that would help the cannabis industry:

"When the curtain finally closes on 2018, it will likely be remembered as the greatest year in cannabis history. To our north, Canada cast aside nine decades of recreational marijuana prohibition and legalized adult-use weed. Although it'll take a few years for growing capacity to be fully ramped up, recreational legalization should add in the neighborhood of $5 billion in annual sales by early next decade. Meanwhile, in the U.S., a handful of states gave the green light to medical or recreational cannabis. There are now 32 medical marijuana-legal states and 10 that allow adult-use pot. We also witnessed the first cannabisderived drug gain approval from the U.S. Food and Drug Administration. Earlier this week, Sen. Cory Gardner (R-Colo.) reintroduced the States Act, which is designed to protect the interests of states with regard to marijuana. In particular, it would recognize that compliant transactions in legalized states aren't considered "trafficking," which would therefore no longer constitute an

216 *McConnell gets $50,000 from pharma after blocking bill to lower drug prices* By Josh Israel AMERICAN INDEPENDENT. February 18, 2020

unlawful transaction by the federal government's definition. Essentially, it would allow states to regulate their own industries without the fear of federal intervention. Why make this move? More than anything, the States Act would open the door to basic banking services for the marijuana industry. If pot companies had access to checking accounts, lines of credit, and loans, they would be able to hire more workers, expand more quickly, reorder supplies with regularity, and move away from a reliance on cash, which is a security concern. Gardner reintroduced the States Act on Monday, Dec. 17, as an amendment to the First Step Act, a criminal justice reform bill that has plenty of support on Capitol Hill and is widely expected to be signed into law. This is a bill that would reduce sentences for nonviolent offenders. By attaching it as an amendment to a larger, popular bill, Gardner hoped to change the way cannabis businesses seek financial services with ease. Of course, the attached amendment needed to first get by Senate Majority Leader Mitch McConnell (R-Ky.). It failed to do so. Despite McConnell spearheading industrial hemp reform via the Farm Bill, which could become a major revenue driver within his home state of Kentucky, McConnell has shunned attempts to reform federal cannabis laws. Disallowing the attached amendment causes Gardner's second attempt to have the States Act signed into law to again come up short. [217]

After taking money from the opiate manufacturers, the leader of the United States Senate will not allow any votes on cannabis reform. Democracy ends with this one man. He also receives donations from liquor companies[218], which are also in direct competition with cannabis. Pharmaceutical companies have a good reason to purchase influence against cannabis legalization. In states that legalized the drug, the use of legal pharmaceutical drugs dropped sharply:

"Research published Wednesday found that states that legalized medical marijuana — which is sometimes recommended for symptoms like chronic pain, anxiety or depression — saw declines in the number of Medicare prescriptions for drugs used to treat those conditions and a dip in spending by Medicare Part D, which covers the cost on prescription medications. Because the prescriptions for drugs like opioid painkillers and antidepressants — and associated Medicare spending on those drugs — fell in states where marijuana could feasibly be used as a replacement, the researchers said it appears likely legalization led to a drop

217 *Mitch McConnell Blocks Marijuana Banking Reform Amendment*. BY Sean Williams. MOTLEY FOOL. Dec 22, 2018
218 *Fueled by their donations, Mitch McConnel pushes special tax break for bourbon industry.* RAND PAUL TRENDOLIZER.

in prescriptions. That point, they said, is strengthened because prescriptions didn't drop for medicines such as blood-thinners, for which marijuana isn't an alternative."[219]

Drug companies are already losing sales. Because the medicinal properties of cannabis are becoming well-known, these companies must shut down legal cannabis, and Donald Trump might be their last hope. He has designed new regulations that keep cannabis illegal, and at the same time, have given them an opportunity to profit off of legal cannabinoid drugs:

"Insys Therapeutics, a pharmaceutical company that was one of the chief financial backers of the opposition to marijuana legalization in Arizona last year, received preliminary approval from the Drug Enforcement Administration this week for Syndros, a synthetic marijuana drug. Insys gave $500,000 last summer to Arizonans for Responsible Drug Policy, the group opposing marijuana legalization in Arizona. The donation amounted to roughly 10 percent of all money raised by the group in an ultimately successful campaign against legalization. Insys was the only pharmaceutical company known to be giving money to oppose legalization last year, according to a Washington Post analysis of campaign finance records. Syndros is a synthetic formulation of THC, the main psychoactive component in the cannabis plant. It was approved by the FDA last summer to treat nausea, vomiting and weight loss in cancer and AIDS patients. The DEA approval places Syndros and its generic formulations in Schedule II of the Controlled Substances Act, indicating a "high potential for abuse." Other Schedule II drugs include cocaine, morphine and many prescription painkillers." [220]

A company that gave money *against* cannabis legalization has developed a drug made from cannabis. This demonstrates extreme hypocrisy. These same companies have given to the Trump reelection effort, and have former employees, and lobbyists in key positions in the White House. They want cannabis to stay illegal, despite public opinion. No President of any political party is brazen enough to move against the will of the voters—except Donald Trump.

---

219 *After Medical Marijuana Legalized, Medicare Prescriptions Drop For Many Drugs*. By Shefali Luthra. NPR.July 6, 2016

220 *A pharma company that spent $500,000 trying to keep pot illegal just got DEA approval for synthetic marijuana*. By Christopher Ingraham. THE WASHINGTON POST.March 24, 2017

CHAPTER 9:
TARGET: CBD

*T*hroughout this country, people have found relief in CBD (cannabidiol), sold throughout this country as a dietary supplement. This cannabinoid does not intoxicate, and fights pain. The top three conditions people use CBD for are relieving stress, reducing pain, and skin conditions[221]. This puts CBD is in serious competition with over the counter, and prescription drugs. This would come to an end, according to regulations just released by the FDA, approved by the Trump Administration.

Everyone should have the right to treat their conditions with a substance that is less expensive than many prescriptions, has less side effects, and has been declared safe by the World Health Organization. The "web" of influence the pharmaceutical industry has on the Trump Administration stretches out to threaten CBD. CBD is technically illegal according to federal laws. The Trump Administration, and the FDA *were* looking the other way—for the moment.

These new rules—basically identical to the new regulations for cannabis research—seek to give control of any patented, cannabinoid combination to the pharmaceutical industry, after being tested by the FDA:

> "It removes from control in schedule V under 21 CFR 1308.15(f) a "drug product in finished dosage formulation that has been approved by the U.S. Food and Drug Administration that contains cannabidiol ...derived from cannabis and no more than 0.1 % (w/w) residual tetrahydrocannabinols." It also removes the import and export controls described in 21 CFR 1312.30(b) over those same substances. It modifies 21 CFR 1308.11(d)

---

221 ***Can CBD improve your health?*** MTL TIMES. TL TIMES. July 23, 2020

(58) by stating that the definition of "Marihuana Extract" is limited to extracts "containing greater than 0.3 percent delta-9-tetrahydrocannabinol on a dry weight basis.[222]"

These new rules will reschedule any extract containing CBD, or other cannabinoids after being tested by the FDA. But THC, and CBD by themselves will continue to be controlled as a Schedule V substance under the 1961 UN Single Convention on Narcotic Drugs, which means they will continue to be placed on Schedule 1 of the CSA. This means the public cannot legally purchase it, with or without a prescription. These rules also mean the public must wait 15 years until new patented drugs go through clinical trials at the FDA, and are approved. After this, the public will pay a higher price for a pharmaceutical drug likely as effective as genuine CBD oil.

Pre-clinical studies indicate both CBD, and THC fight cancer. But after these new rules are fully implemented according to the law, people who have cancer now will not have access to this oil anymore. As the closure of dispensaries, the President could use government agencies, and current laws to levy fines, causing all CBD to be pulled from the shelves. Racketeering drug laws can be used against these businesses right now.

In a recent clinical trial, a CBD based prescription prolonged the lives of brain cancer patients:

> "Findings from a new study examining human and canine brain cancer cells suggest that cannabidiol could be a useful therapy for a difficult-to-treat brain cancer. Cannabidiol, or CBD, is a non-psychoactive chemical compound derived from marijuana. The study looked at glioblastoma, an often-deadly form of brain cancer that grows and spreads very quickly. Even with major advancements in treatment, survival rates for this cancer have not improved significantly. "Further research and treatment options are urgently needed for patients afflicted by brain cancer," said Chase Gross, a student in the Doctor of Veterinary Medicine/Master of Science program at Colorado State University. "Our work shows that CBD has the potential to provide an effective, synergistic glioblastoma therapy option and that it should continue to be vigorously studied."[223]

Despite this fantastic news, it will take years for applications to be filed, tests to be run, and physicians to be taught—before this will be used as a cancer treatment. Cancer patients can't wait while all of these studies are conducted. A woman with breast cancer is running out of time:

---

222 Implementation of the agriculture improvement act of 2018. FEDERAL REGISTER.

223 *Study shows that CBD isolate and extract can slow growth and kill cancer cells* NEWSWISE April 27, 2020

"CBD is in our lattes, moisturizers, and chocolates, but what about its use in a hospital setting instead of your local café or beauty store? Although more study is needed, research suggests that CBD may have the potential to help relieve certain side effects of chemotherapy. CBD is short for cannabidiol, which is one of the many compounds found in cannabis and hemp. Unlike tetrahydrocannabinol (THC), it's non-psychoactive. Manufacturers have found a way to separate CBD from the plants, and the Agriculture Improvement Act of 2018 (aka the Farm Bill) legalized hemp-derived CBD that contains no more than 0.3% THC and is made from hemp grown by licensed producers. (That's why you've seen so many CBD products recently.) But so far, the Food and Drug Administration has only approved one form of CBD: Epidiolex, a drug containing a purified marijuana-derived form of CBD, which is used for preventing seizures caused by rare forms of epilepsy."[224]

CBD could treat many different cancers, but the evidence favors THC, which this Administration also wants to tightly control. If the President *really* believes that THC causes a drop in IQ, schizophrenia, and violence, any actions taken against this drug would not be self-serving. Although misguided, any actions against THC would be taken with the best intentions. This however, might not be the case.

CBD does not intoxicate. It is not addictive. There would be no reason to demand this drug remain on Schedule 1, unless some of the people in cabinet positions, with ties the pharmaceutical industry *suggest it*. In any case, these new regulations will work for their benefit.

President Trump's Anti-CBD Actions

President Trump's pick for Drug Czar, Tom Marino, voted against removing restrictions on CBD oil[225], as the new CBD regulations perpetuate, approved by President Trump. The Trump Administration has also banned military vets from using CBD:

"The Drug Warrior takeover of the Trump administration now

---

224 *The Miracle That Is CBD, Might Help Breast Cancer Patients Too* By Erika W. Smith. YAHOO NEWS. October 10, 2019

225 ...he voted against a measure to allow Veterans Affairs doctors to recommend medical marijuana to their patients, as well as against a separate measure to loosen federal restrictions on hemp, a non-psychoactive variant of the cannabis plant with potential industrial applications. Those votes place Marino well to the right of dozens of his Republican House colleagues who supported the measures. He also voted against a measure that would loosen some restrictions on CBD oil, a non-psychoactive derivative of the cannabis plant that holds promise for treating severe forms of childhood epilepsy. THE CANNABIST

seems complete with the ban on CBD use by the military because it might interfere with marijuana testing. The MarijuanaMoment. net website reported the new policy calling it "little-noticed," which is an accurate but ironic description of what should have been widely announced, if it was meant to inform members of both the active duty and reserve military about something so important. The Department of Defense (DOD) announced the new policy in February, banning all active and reserve service members from using hemp products, including CBD."[226]

If members of the military could use CBD for pain instead of opiates, this could save lives. But the President doesn't care. He is so concerned with keeping CBD on Schedule 1, even *shampoos* containing CBD are banned:

"The Navy is expanding its CBD and hemp ban for sailors and marines to cover topical products like shampoos and soaps derived from the federally legal crop, going beyond a previous prohibition focused on consumable preparations such as oils and tinctures. In its new Friday memo, the Navy clarified that "use" of banned products "includes the use of topical products containing hemp, such as shampoos, conditioners, lotions, lip balms, or soaps.""[227]

According to current laws, members of the military can consume alcohol, take prescription opiates, or anti-psychotics for PTSD with no problem, as long as a product doesn't contain even *a little* THC. These men can fight in wars, lose their lives for their country—but even a *little* THC is unacceptable to this Administration.

CBD is Technically Illegal

The logical reason for Trump's strict CBD military ban is it goes against his plan to keep it illegal—and pull it from the shelves after his reelection. Right now, CBD products break Federal laws:

"It fits into a new conception of health, wellness and functional foods that includes the nonintoxicating benefits of this chemical compound without the psychoactive THC found in marijuana. But at the federal level, CBD in food and drink is still illegal. The Federal Food, Drug & Cosmetic Act prohibits adding even approved drugs to human or animal food in interstate commerce. The 2018 Farm Bill legalized hemp, but the legal status of hemp-derived cannabidiol remains in limbo. This is largely because

226 *Trump's Ban on CBD for the Military Echoes Drug War, Anti-Hemp Oil Hysteria*. By Richard Cowan. LA WEEKLY. July 6, 2020

227 *Navy Bans Hemp Shampoo For Sailors And Marines As Part Of Broader CBD Prohibition*. By Kyle Jaeger. MARIJUANA MOMENT. July 27, 2020

CBD can be derived from hemp or cannabis, but if a hemp plant contains more than 0.3 percent THC (the active "high" ingredient in marijuana) it is then technically a "marijuana" plant." [228]

Although CBD is sold on shelves of stores throughout this nation, the government has been looking the other way. Although Hemp was made legal in the farm bill, it is the position of the FDA that all cannabinoid extractions are currently *illegal*:

> "The Farm Bill also created regulations for hemp farmers, which means, "that any cannabinoid—a set of chemical compounds found in the cannabis plant—that is derived from hemp will be legal, if and only if that hemp is produced in a manner consistent with the Farm Bill, associated federal regulations, association state regulations, and by a licensed grower," according to the Brookings Institute, a non-profit public policy organization. In other words, if a CBD product contains the legal amount of THC but wasn't grown by a licensed producer according to federal regulations, it's still illegal. The day the Farm Bill was signed into law, the US Food and Drug Administration (FDA) released a statement clarifying that Congress had "explicitly preserved the agency's current authority to regulate products containing cannabis or cannabis-derived compounds under the Federal Food, Drug, and Cosmetic Act (FD&C Act) and section 351 of the Public Health Service Act." Because CBD is also an approved prescription drug (Epidiolex), the FDA still considers CBD a drug ingredient, which means it cannot be marketed and sold as a dietary supplement with therapeutic properties (or even shipped across state lines) without first going through the FDA's drug approval process -- regardless of whether the products are derived from hemp."[229]

After the 2014 Farm Bill was passed, and CBD began to be sold in the stores, the DEA continued to treat it as a Schedule 1 substance. That was vague in the law at that time, but has been clarified now. CBD *is* a Schedule 1 substance. The DEA raided businesses, causing an uproar. So, what did the government do? They added a new regulation in the federal code that *kept CBD technically illegal*:

> "The DEA code for marijuana is 7360, while the new marijuana extract code is 7350. Some observers believe the rule change could mean increased federal interference in the hemp industry. But the executive director of the Hemp Industry Association,

228 ***CBD is still illegal in the US. So why is it everywhere?*** By the Washington Post. THE MERCURY NEWS. June 25, 2019
229 *Is CBD Legal?* By Danielle Kosecki. CNET. Aug. 2, 2019

Eric Steenstra, said the rule doesn't do anything new – since CBD products are already illegal – other than give CBD oils and other extracted products another federal government tracking code.....The rule also said that marijuana extracts will continue to be treated as Schedule I controlled substances, even if they are CBD products derived from hemp, which by federal definition contains less than 0.3% THC. The DEA said that even if THC and other federally prohibited cannabinoids could theoretically be removed from CBD products, it hasn't been done, and therefore CBD products are federally illegal."[230]

This "new drug code" uses a legalistic trick. It was established a few months before President Trump took office, yet he has whole-heartedly embraced it. Of course, President Trump is not the only problem. *Both parties* have been corrupted by pharmaceutical money, and might take "suggestions" from lobbyists, without considering every ramification. The DEA under President Obama, and Chuck Rosenberg created this new rule to keep CBD illegal, but not Hemp:

"The new drug code (7350) established in the Final Rule does not include materials or products that are excluded from the definition of marijuana set forth in the Controlled Substances Act (CSA).1 The new drug code includes only those extracts that fall within the CSA definition of marijuana. If a product consisted solely of parts of the cannabis plant excluded from the CSA definition of marijuana, such product would not be included in the new drug code (7350) or in the drug code for marijuana (7360). As explained in the Final Rule, the creation of this new drug code was primarily intended to give DEA more precise accounting to assist the agency in carrying out its obligations to provide certain reports required by U.S. treaty obligations. Because the Final Rule did not add any substance to the schedules that was not already controlled, and did not change the schedule of any substance, it was not a scheduling action under 21 U.S.C. §§ 811 and 812. The new drug code is a subset of what has always been included in the CSA definition of marijuana. By creating a new drug code for marijuana extract, the Final Rule divides into more descriptive pieces the materials, compounds, mixtures, and preparations that fall within the CSA definition of marijuana. Both drug code 7360 (marijuana) and new drug code 7350 (marijuana extract) are limited to that which falls within the CSA definition of marijuana. Because recent public inquiries that DEA has received following the publication of the Final Rule suggest there may be some misunderstanding about the source

---

230 *DEA rule change sparks concern on marijuana extracts*. HEMP INDUSTRY DAILY. December 14, 2016

of cannabinoids in the cannabis plant, we also note the following botanical considerations. As the scientific literature indicates, cannabinoids, such as tetrahydrocannabinols (THC), cannabinols (CBN) and cannabidiols (CBD), are found in the parts of the cannabis plant that fall within the CSA definition of marijuana, such as the flowering tops, resin, and leaves.2 According to the scientific literature, cannabinoids are not found in the parts of the cannabis plant that are excluded from the CSA definition of marijuana, except for trace amounts (typically, only parts per million)3 that may be found where small quantities of resin adhere to the surface of seeds and mature stalk.4 Thus, based on the scientific literature, it is not practical to produce extracts that contain more than trace amounts of cannabinoids using only the parts of the cannabis plant that are excluded from the CSA definition of marijuana, such as oil from the seeds. The industrial processes used to clean cannabis seeds and produce seed oil would likely further diminish any trace amounts of cannabinoids that end up in the finished product. However, as indicated above, if a product, such as oil from cannabis seeds, consisted solely of parts of the cannabis plant excluded from the CSA definition of marijuana, such product would not be included in the new drug code (7350) or in the drug code for marijuana (7360), even if it contained trace amounts of cannabinoids."[231]

This New Rule was created under Chuck Rosenberg, who President Trump retained to head the DEA. This rules defines CBD oil in a special manner, to place it on Schedule 1 of the CSA—but not Hemp. This legalistic trick has caused confusion throughout the Hemp industry:

"For practical purposes, all extracts that contain CBD will also contain at least small amounts of other cannabinoids.[1] However, if it were possible to produce from the cannabis plant an extract that contained only CBD and no other cannabinoids, such an extract would fall within the new drug code 7350. In view of this comment, the regulatory text accompanying new drug code 7350 has been modified slightly to make clear that it includes cannabis extracts that contain only one cannabinoid." It would be reasonable to construe this as DEA criminalizing CBD. The Hemp Industries Association (HIA), Summerland, CA challenges DEA's notion that CBD was under Schedule I prior to this Final Rule and states that they lack the authority to change the legal status of CBD, which can only done by Congress of the Attorney General. "The ruling is based on an incorrect and incomplete understanding of how CBD is derived from the cannabis plant,"

<hr>

231 ***Clarification of the New Drug Code (7350) for Marijuana Extract.*** DEA DIVERSION.

explains HIA. "While CBD may be derived from forms of cannabis that contain high amounts of THC...CBD may also be produced from industrial hemp plants that meet the legal standards of less than 0.3% THC by dry weight, and which may be cultivated in 32 states in the U.S. per Sec. 7606 of the Farm Bill, the Legitimacy of Industrial Hemp Research amendment."[232]

Investments made throughout the Hemp industry will be lost, if the government controls CBD as a prescription drug—as stated in these new rules. Unless CBD is reclassified as a supplement, only products made from the seeds, stalk, and stem of Hemp will be legal to sell in stores.

The man Trump chose to keep as head of the DEA made this statement about Cannabis:

"If you want me to say that marijuana's not dangerous, I'm not going to say that because I think it is. Do I think it's as dangerous as heroin? Probably not. I'm not an expert."[233]

Several observations should be made about Mr Rosenberg's statement. First, as head of the DRUG Enforcement agency, shouldn't he be an expert in drugs? Secondly, anyone who has conducted *any* research knows THC is not anywhere near as dangerous as heroin, or alcohol either. Thirdly, President Trump kept him on as head of the DEA, *after he made this statement*. If you were President, would you keep a man in this job, that believes this? Anyone who really believes cannabis is as dangerous as heroin, cannot possibly be fair about cannabis laws. Lastly, this thinking is right in line with the Memo circulated by President Trump's legal team at the DEA. The President believes in order to keep international obligations, cannabis must be regulated *as opium*. Mr Rosenberg is an accomplished lawyer, and likely had a hand in writing this convoluted, legalistic rule. He tweeted this statement at the time the rule was announced:

"Maybe you can grow hemp. But if you try to extract the CBD oil, the DEA will consider it a federal crime."[234]

The fact that the Trump Administration kept Mr Rosenberg in his position of power speaks volumes about the President's true intentions. His refusal to reclassify CBD as a supplement proves he agrees with Rosenberg on this position. Rosenberg also spoke out *against* opposition to the law that "tied the DEA's hands" against opiate manufacturers:

"The article reported on internal dissent within the DEA about this

232 *DEA Issues New Drug Code Causing Confusion About CBD's Legal Status*. WHOLE FOODS MAGAZINE. December 20, 2016

233 *New Drug Enforcement Agency Chief Says He's "Not an Expert" on Drugs*. By Jack Moore. GQ MAGAZINE. July 31, 2015

234 *CBD becomes a dangerous substance in the USA*. CANNABIS MAGAZINE. December 15, 2016

legislation and quoted Joseph Rannazzisi, a former DEA deputy assistant administrator, as saying of Congress: "They are taking the word of industry rather than the government's expert in diversion control." In her letter, Chu explained that in her meeting with Rosenberg last year, she learned that the DEA had had been consulted by legislators about the bill and that the agency felt the "legislation was unnecessary." "[Rosenberg] reiterated that it was not the agency's position that this bill would interfere with the agency efforts to stop harmful opioids from entering our communities," Chu added."[235]

No we know Mr. Rosenberg was wrong. The law did impede on the ability of his agency to do it's job, and helped create the "opiate epidemic." After Mr Rosenberg left the DEA, he joined a firm that represents multinational corporations, including pharmaceutical companies, *Crowell and Moring*. So, although circumstantial, these connections should be considered. Rosenberg made decisions *against* CBD, and in favor of opiates. Furthermore, the man President Trump chose as his replacement also believes cannabis is as bad as heroin. Fortunately, he was not confirmed.

FDA Warnings About CBD

The FDA has approved only one CBD product, a prescription drug to treat two rare, severe forms of epilepsy. Here are the warnings the FDA has posted on it's website:

> • *It is currently illegal to market CBD by adding it to a food or labeling it as a dietary supplement.*
> • *The FDA has seen only limited data about CBD safety and these data point to real risks that need to be considered before taking CBD for any reason.*
> • *Some CBD products are being marketed with unproven medical claims and are of unknown quality.*
> • *The FDA will continue to update the public as it learns more about CBD.*
> *CBD has the potential to harm you, and harm can happen even before you become aware of it.*

So far these FDA warnings are quite benign. But then we read:

> • *CBD can cause liver injury.*

This claim is based on a study that used faulty methods, as the "THC Monkey Mask study." Researchers fed mice up to *one quarter of their body*

---

235 *Congresswoman demands investigation into law that stymied DEA on opioid enforcement.* By Benjamin Oreskes. LA TIMES. October 19, 2017

weight of CBD, then recorded liver disease:

> "Many experts have weighed in on the mouse study and its flaws. The main problem with this study is that the initial dose chosen for the investigation was equivalent to 20 mgs of CBD per kg of body weight, which is analogous to those used in clinical trials for the FDA-approved CBD epilepsy drug, Epidiolex. This dose would be equal to a 150 pound human taking over 1300 mgs of CBD! To put that into perspective, the typical dose of CBD oil users is somewhere in the range of 10 to 80 mgs per day, with slightly higher doses for therapeutic issues or "flare-ups". As we can see, this study does not mimic the typical usage patterns of most CBD consumers. The study itself states that their dosages "is not applicable to most real-life scenarios", but goes on to say that "it does provide critical information regarding the potential consequences of CBD overdose."[236]

This claim is based on bad science. No one takes this much CBD. Forcing these mice to consume one quarter of body weight in CBD proves these researchers set out to find something bad. Any drug in excess can damage the liver—from Tylenol to alcohol. So, the Food and Drug Administration posts information based on a debunked study, as evidence against the safety of CBD. Of course, paid advisors who worked at the FDA have worked for companies against legalization of CBD.

> *"CBD can affect how other drugs you are taking work, potentially causing serious side effects."*

This statement is true, but no reason to prohibit it's sale, or use. Over the counter supplements, and other pharmaceutical drugs can affect how a prescription works. Everyone should inform their physician of anything they take (unless is suspected the Physician will deny treatment for cannabis use.) Alcohol can also interfere with some medications. This is no reason to prohibit CBD.

> • *Use of CBD with alcohol or other drugs that slow brain activity, such as those used to treat anxiety, panic, stress, or sleep disorders, increases the risk of sedation and drowsiness, which can lead to injuries.*

This statement is also true. Yet again, so can many medications, *and alcohol.*

> • *Male reproductive toxicity, or damage to fertility in males or*

---

236 ***Does CBD Cause Liver Damage? Why You Shouldn't Worry.*** TESSERA NATURALS. April 30, 2020_

*male offspring of women who have been exposed, has been
reported in studies of animals exposed to CBD.*

The FDA is confused. In mice, a THC/CBD *combination* does lower sperm count:

"Sperm morphology was studied in hybrid mice of genotype (C57BL X C3H)F1 following treatment with specific cannabinoids. Mice were treated for 5 consecutive days with the specific cannabinoid; 35 days after the last treatment, epididymal sperm were scored in the light microscope and assessed in the scanning electron microscope. The animals treated with delta9-tetrahydrocannabinol (delta9-THC) and cannabinol (CBN) had a statistically higher incidence of abnormal sperm than the controls. The incidence of abnormal sperm in the animals treated with cannabidiol (CBD) was not statistically different from the control value. The relative toxicity of the cannabinoids in these studies was delta9-THC greater than CBN greater than CBD. Normal sperm have a smooth kidney-shaped head with a prominent hook; abnormal sperm have shapes which include heads without hooks, banana-shaped heads, amorphous heads and folded heads."[237]

According to this study, a combination THC/CBD does lower sperm count up to 25%, but *CBD alone does nothing*. Yet, their statement is *more* than false, but uses extremely old data. The FDA ignores newer studies that indicate no change in sperm count:

Forget the mellow slacker image -- pot smoking might actually make men more potent. Men who've smoked marijuana appear to have significantly higher sperm concentrations than those who've never given it a try, a new study reports. There's also a potential link between pot use and testosterone, said senior researcher Dr. Jorge Chavarro. He's an associate professor of nutrition and epidemiology at the Harvard T.H. Chan School of Public Health in Boston. "With increasing use of marijuana, there was a positive association with serum testosterone levels," Chavarro said. "More marijuana, higher testosterone levels."[238]

CBD can cause side effects that you might notice. These side effects should improve when CBD is stopped or when the amount used is reduced.• Changes in alertness, most commonly

237 **Effects of cannabinoids on sperm morphology**. PHARMACOLOGY. PUBMED. 1979
238 **Could Smoking a Little Pot Raise Sperm Levels?** By Dennis Thompson. WEBMD. February 6, 2019

experienced as somnolence (drowsiness or sleepiness).

This is true. But again, is no reason to prohibit it's use. A number of over the counter medications, and vitamin supplements cause drowsiness, including:

> • Diphenhydramine (Benadryl, Aleve PM, others).
> Diphenhydramine is a sedating antihistamine. Side effects
> might include daytime drowsiness, dry mouth, blurred vision,
> constipation and urinary retention.
> • Doxylamine succinate (Unisom SleepTabs). Doxylamine is also
> a sedating antihistamine. Side effects are similar to those of
> diphenhydramine.
> • Melatonin. The hormone melatonin helps control your natural
> sleep-wake cycle. Some research suggests that melatonin
> supplements might be helpful in treating jet lag or reducing
> the time it takes to fall asleep — although the effect is typically
> mild. Side effects can include headaches and daytime sleepiness.
> • Valerian. Supplements made from this plant are sometimes
> taken as sleep aids. Although a few studies indicate some
> therapeutic benefit, other studies haven't found the same
> benefits. Valerian generally doesn't appear to cause side
> effects.[239]

The FDA does not object to any of these over the counter medications, or herbal supplements that also cause drowsiness. The FDA is merely posting excuses to sway public opinion from treating their illnesses on their own with CBD. After 15 years of testing, and the drug companies control it, then it will be ok.

> • *Gastrointestinal distress, most commonly experienced as*
> *diarrhea and/or decreased appetite.*

Taking too much CBD oil can cause diarrhea as a side effect. Yet again, this is no cause from keeping if from the American public. Many other drugs can cause diarrhea, including these heartburn medications:

> "Drugs used to treat heartburn and stomach ulcers, such as
> omeprazole (Prilosec), esomeprazole (Nexium), lansoprazole
> (Prevacid), rabeprazole (AcipHex), pantoprazole (Protonix),
> cimetidine (Tagamet), ranitidine (Zantac), and nizatidine (Axid)."[240]

The FDA has *no problem* with any of these medications that cause diarrhea as a side effect—*except one, Zantac.* It was approved, but pulled from

---

239 *Sleep aids: Understand over-the-counter options.* MAYO CLINIC
240 *Drug-induced diarrhea* MEDLINE PLUS https://medlineplus.gov/ency/article/000293.htm

the market because it can potentially cause cancer. And of course, antibiotics cause diarrhea, as well as alcohol abuse. This should never be a reason to prohibit a substance.

> • *Changes in mood, most commonly experienced as irritability and agitation.* (All FDA warnings from: ***What You Need to Know (And What We're Working to Find Out) About Products Containing Cannabis or Cannabis-derived Compounds, Including CBD***[241])

Once again, the FDA is not being completely honest. This claim has been debunked:

> "Introduction: This literature survey aims to extend the comprehensive survey performed by Bergamaschi et al. in 2011 on cannabidiol (CBD) safety and side effects. Apart from updating the literature, this article focuses on clinical studies and CBD potential interactions with other drugs. Results: In general, the often described favorable safety profile of CBD in humans was confirmed and extended by the reviewed research. The majority of studies were performed for treatment of epilepsy and psychotic disorders. Here, the most commonly reported side effects were tiredness, diarrhea, and changes of appetite/weight. In comparison with other drugs, used for the treatment of these medical conditions, CBD has a better side effect profile. This could improve patients' compliance and adherence to treatment. CBD is often used as adjunct therapy. Therefore, more clinical research is warranted on CBD action on hepatic enzymes, drug transporters, and interactions with other drugs and to see if this mainly leads to positive or negative effects, for example, reducing the needed clobazam doses in epilepsy and therefore clobazam's side effects. Conclusion: This review also illustrates that some important toxicological parameters are yet to be studied, for example, if CBD has an effect on hormones. Additionally, more clinical trials with a greater number of participants and longer chronic CBD administration are still lacking."[242]

This study honestly addresses this claim. Irritability reported among CBD users occurred in clinical trials with *epilepsy, and psychiatric patients*. This sample is not representative of the general population, and is inaccurate for obvious reasons. With most forms of epilepsy, CBD greatly reduces seizures, but

241 ***What You Need to Know (And What We're Working to Find Out) About Products Containing Cannabis or Cannabis-derived Compounds, Including CBD***
242 ***An Update on Safety and Side Effects of Cannabidiol: A Review of Clinical Data and Relevant Animal Studies.*** CANNABIS AND CANNABINOID RESEARCH. PUBMED. July 1, 2017

does not eliminate them. After a seizure, someone who suffers from epilepsy can feel depressed, or agitated for days:

> "Many recent epidemiological studies have found the prevalence of depression and anxiety to be higher in people with epilepsy (PWE) than in people without epilepsy. Furthermore, people with depression or anxiety have been more likely to suffer from epilepsy than those without depression or anxiety. Almost one-third of PWE suffer from depression and anxiety, which is similar to the prevalence of drug-refractory epilepsy. Various brain areas, including the frontal, temporal, and limbic regions, are associated with the biological pathogenesis of depression in PWE."[243]

Depression and anxiety are symptoms of epilepsy. And of course, everyone knows psychiatric patients are anxious and depressed. These researchers overlooked this simple fact, and got paid for it. Therefore, this claim by this FDA is based on studies based on a subset of the population known to have these problems.

Statement by the World Health Organization

As the FDA is making these claims against CBD, the World Health Organization has investigated this substance, and found it to be completely safe:

> "At its 40th Meeting the ECDD considered a critical review of cannabidiol and recommended that preparations considered to be pure cannabidiol should not be scheduled within the International Drug Control Conventions. Cannabidiol is found in cannabis and cannabis resin but does not have psychoactive properties and has no potential for abuse and no potential to produce dependence. It does not have significant ill-effects."[244]

Despite this recommendation by the World Health Organization, the European Union has announced it will vote *against* removing CBD from Schedule V of the 1961 Single Convention on Narcotic Drugs:

> "The executive branch of the European Union is changing its stance on how EU countries should vote on the World Health Organization's cannabis scheduling changes in December, Hemp Industry Daily has learned. The development comes on the heels of the European Commission announcing its preliminary view

243 ***Depression and Anxiety in People with Epilepsy***. JOURNAL OF CLINICAL NEUROLOGY. PUBMED July 3, 2014

244 ***Annex 1- Extract from the Report of the 41st Expert Committee on Drug Dependence: Cannabis and cannabis-related substances***. WORLD HEALTH ORGANIZATION. posted by MARIJUANA BUISNESS DAILY.

that CBD extracted from the flowering tops of the Cannabis sativa L. plant should be considered a narcotic under a 1961 United Nations treaty. If the Commission's new stance is formally adopted, hemp-derived CBD would no longer be considered food, would fall outside the scope of the bloc's novel food regulation and could be banned from the EU market....While the commission's "treat CBD as narcotic" stance is itself not shocking, "it is extremely puzzling why they have come forward with this position now," said Eveline Van Keymeulen, a Paris-based attorney at Allen & Overy. According to Van Keymeulen, precedent for the commission's view of CBD can be found in the European Commission's proposal for how EU countries should vote on the WHO cannabis scheduling recommendations this December. "What is very surprising is the timing," said Van Keymeulen. "We've had novel food status for two years, and after interacting with so many member states and authorities, and updating the [Novel Food] Catalog several times, what they are doing now is totally backpedaling." "No one really knows why the European Union wants to ban hemp extracts at all – which would mean the definitive end of the hemp food industry except for hemp seeds," said Kai-Friedrich Niermann, an attorney based in Germany who specializes in CBD and cannabis regulations. "That can't be the solution and that can't be the future."[245]

President Trump was likely behind the European Union's change of heart. Remember, the basic argument of this Administration against the legalization of cannabis, and CBD, is based on a strict interpretion of international treaties. Of course, these rules were written over 40 years ago, by men who also received pharmaceutical donations. It cannot be coincidental that suddenly the European Union is also abiding by a strict interpretion of these treaties.

The 2018 Farm Bill

The 2018 farm only removed some obstacles facing the CBD industry. However, after it was passed, the FDA reiterated that CBD was illegal:

"The passage of the 2018 Farm Bill has led to the misperception that all products made from or containing hemp, including those made with CBD, are now legal to sell in interstate commerce. The result has been that storefronts and online retailers have flooded the market with these products, many with unsubstantiated

---

245 ***EU Commission revises stance on WHO cannabis scheduling vote as it leans toward CBD as a narcotic.*** By Monica Raymut. HEMP INDUSTRY DAILY. July 30, 2020

therapeutic claims. FDA has seen CBD appear in a wide variety of products including foods, dietary supplements, veterinary products, and cosmetics.. As this new market emerges, we have seen substantial interest from industry, consumers, and Congress. However, in the midst of the excitement and innovation, FDA's role remains the same: to protect and promote the public health. At present, any CBD food or purported dietary supplement products in interstate commerce is in violation of the FD&C Act due to the statutory provisions discussed above."[246]

It continues to be illegal to sell CBD as a dietary supplement:

Can THC or CBD products be sold as dietary supplements? A. No. Based on available evidence, FDA has concluded that THC and CBD products are excluded from the dietary supplement definition under section 201(ff)(3)(B) of the FD&C Act [21 U.S.C. § 321(ff)(3)(B)]. Under that provision, if a substance (such as THC or CBD) is an active ingredient in a drug product that has been approved under section 505 of the FD&C Act [21 U.S.C. § 355], or has been authorized for investigation as a new drug for which substantial clinical investigations have been instituted and for which the existence of such investigations has been made public, then products containing that substance are excluded from the definition of a dietary supplement. FDA considers a substance to be "authorized for investigation as a new drug" if it is the subject of an Investigational New Drug application (IND) that has gone into effect. Under FDA's regulations (21 CFR 312.2), unless a clinical investigation meets the limited criteria in that regulation, an IND is required for all clinical investigations of products that are subject to section 505 of the FD&C Act. There is an exception to section 201(ff)(3)(B) if the substance was "marketed as" a dietary supplement or as a conventional food before the drug was approved or before the new drug investigations were authorized, as applicable. However, based on available evidence, FDA has concluded that this is not the case for THC or CBD."[247]

Here is a statement made at the time by the former head of the FDA, Scott Gottlieb:

"For Immediate Release: December 20, 2018 Statement From: Commissioner of Food and Drugs - Food and Drug Administration

246 *Hemp Production and the 2018 Farm Bill*. FOOD AND DRUG ADMINISTRATION. July 25, 2019
247 *FDA Regulation of Cannabis and Cannabis-Derived Products, Including Cannabidiol (CBD)*. FOOD AND DRUG ADMINISTRATION. August 3, 2020

Scott Gottlieb M.D. Today, the Agriculture Improvement Act of 2018 was signed into law. Among other things, this new law changes certain federal authorities relating to the production and marketing of hemp, defined as cannabis (Cannabis sativa L.), and derivatives of cannabis with extremely low (less than 0.3 percent on a dry weight basis) concentrations of the psychoactive compound delta-9-tetrahydrocannabinol (THC). These changes include removing hemp from the Controlled Substances Act, which means that it will no longer be an illegal substance under federal law. Just as important for the FDA and our commitment to protect and promote the public health is what the law didn't change: Congress explicitly preserved the agency's current authority to regulate products containing cannabis or cannabis-derived compounds under the Federal Food, Drug, and Cosmetic Act (FD&C Act) and section 351 of the Public Health Service Act. In doing so, Congress recognized the agency's important public health role with respect to all the products it regulates. This allows the FDA to continue enforcing the law to protect patients and the public while also providing potential regulatory pathways for products containing cannabis and cannabis-derived compounds. We're aware of the growing public interest in cannabis and cannabis-derived products, including cannabidiol (CBD). This increasing public interest in these products makes it even more important with the passage of this law for the FDA to clarify its regulatory authority over these products. In short, we treat products containing cannabis or cannabis-derived compounds as we do any other FDA-regulated products — meaning they're subject to the same authorities and requirements as FDA-regulated products containing any other substance. This is true regardless of the source of the substance, including whether the substance is derived from a plant that is classified as hemp under the Agriculture Improvement Act. ...In view of the proliferation of products containing cannabis or cannabis-derived substances, the FDA will advance new steps to better define our public health obligations in this area. We'll also continue to closely scrutinize products that could pose risks to consumers. Where we believe consumers are being put at risk, the FDA will warn consumers and take enforcement actions... We'll take enforcement action needed to protect public health against companies illegally selling cannabis and cannabis-derived products that can put consumers at risk and are being marketed in violation of the FDA's authorities...It should also be noted that some foods are derived from parts of the hemp plant that may not contain CBD or THC, meaning that their addition to foods might not raise the same issues as the addition of drug ingredients like CBD and THC. We are able to advance the lawful marketing of three such ingredients today. We are announcing that the agency has completed our evaluation of three Generally Recognized as Safe (GRAS) notices related to hulled hemp seeds, hemp seed protein and hemp seed oil and that the agency had no questions regarding the company's conclusion that the use of such products as described in the notices is safe. Therefore, these products can be legally marketed in human foods for these uses without food additive approval, provided they comply with all other requirements and do not make disease treatment claims."[248]

Even after leaving the FDA, Dr Gottlieb continued to state that CBD products are illegal:

"The cannabidiol droplets you may be adding into your brunch cocktail are not actually legal, former FDA Commissioner Scott Gottlieb warned on CNBC on Friday. CBD is a compound found in the cannabis plant that's boomed in the retail industry in the past year, with many touting its supposed stress-relieving benefits despite limited evidence. Coffee shops, bars and restaurants have rushed to cash in on adding CBD to foods and beverages. However, the Food and Drug Administration is looking to put a stop to that, citing safety concerns. "You can't just put it in the food supply," said Gottlieb, who left the FDA in April. "Right now, all the CBD is illegal that's being put into food or dietary supplements." Gottlieb, a resident fellow at the right-leaning American Enterprise Institute, is also a physician who consults for and invests in biopharmaceutical companies. He joined Pfizer's board of directors earlier this summer."[249]

The same man who warned us about CBD being illegal, consults for bio-pharmaceutical companies, and joined Pfizer after he left his post. These companies have a vested interest in marketing CBD and THC as pain killers, which would be unprofitable if people continue to have legal access.

Regulatory barrier

There have been several attempts to persuade President Trump to remove CBD from Schedule 1, but to no avail. Seven Hemp organizations

---

248 *FDA Responds to Three GRAS Notices for Hemp Seed-Derived Ingredients for Use in Human Food*. FOOD AND DRUG ADMINISTRATION. December 20, 2018
249 *Former FDA chief warns consumers that all forms of CBD in food is actually illegal*. By Jessica Bursztynsky. CNBC. August 9, 2019

delivered a letter to the President:

> "Seven hemp organizations on Tuesday wrote a letter to President Donald Trump, thanking him for supporting farmers and stating his administration could help resolve a "regulatory barrier" facing the CBD industry. The hemp industry has experienced tremendous growth since passage of the 2018 Farm Bill, with domestic hemp production growing from 25,500 acres in 2017 to 78,000 acres in 2018 to 511,442 acres in 2019, according to the letter. Citing Hemp Business Journal, the groups reported U.S. sales of hemp products are projected to reach $2.6 billion by 2022, up from $820 million in 2018. "The domestic hemp industry is barely 1 year old, and the projected numbers on what our nascent industry can produce are impressive," the organizations wrote. Despite removing hemp and its derivatives from the Controlled Substances Act (CSA), the 2018 Farm Bill preserved FDA's authority to regulate certain cannabis-derived products. And while FDA has been exploring potential regulatory pathways for CBD in conventional food and dietary supplements, many hemp and supplement groups have grown frustrated over lack of any rules or guidance."[250]

Their appeal to President Trump has fallen on deaf ears. No attempt has been made by this Administration to remove CBD from schedule 1, or to reclassify it as a dietary supplement—as several congressional leaders called for:

> "... in addition to regulating pharmaceuticals, the FDA is responsible for controlling additives to food, beverages, and dietary supplements. The excitement surrounding CBD has always been the idea of incorporating the substance into a variety of foods and beverages. In fact, a handful of brand-name companies, including Mondelez International, had tinkered with the idea of creating CBD-infused foods or beverages. However, the FDA has poured cold water on what's been a red-hot industry. After months of review, the FDA laid down the hammer on CBD enthusiasts in a Nov. 25 consumer update. Without providing any concrete guidance, the FDA stated the following: CBD has the potential to harm you. CBD can cause side effects that you might not notice. There are many important aspects of CBD that we just don't know. In effect, the FDA doesn't view CBD as a safe substance, at least not at this time." Congress and the FDA May Square Off Over CBD A new bill introduced in the House would

---

250 ***Hemp groups: Trump could help resolve FDA CBD barrier.*** CANNABINOID INDUSTRY ASSOCIATION

reclassify cannabidiol as a dietary supplement."[251]

A bill was introduced in Congress to reclassify CBD as a dietary supplement:

> "A battle may be brewing between lawmakers and the FDA over CBD However, the FDA's decision to keep CBD out of food, beverages, and dietary supplements for the time being may not be an end-all for the industry. This past week, on Jan. 15, a bipartisan group of lawmakers in the House of Representatives introduced H.R. 5587, a bill that would amend the federal Food, Drug, and Cosmetic Act to classify hemp-derived CBD as a dietary supplement. With CBD products being lumped into the same category as vitamins, the FDA would be required to allow them onto store shelves without the testing that's required of pharmaceutical products, if the bill becomes law."[252]

So far, no bill has passed to reclassify CBD, and is unlikely—considering the position of this Administration, and the people with ties to the pharmaceutical industry he has placed throughout our government. Furthermore, the entire premise of this Administration's regulatory scheme is based on a strict interpretation of international treaties. Classifying CBD as a supplement would violate these treaties.

HHS Petition

As Congress debates reclassifying CBD, another government agency has petitioned the DEA to reschedule it, *and failed.* Assistant Secretary of Health, Brett Giroir made this petition in 2018:

> "Pursuant to the Controlled Substances Act (CSA), U.S.C. §811 (b), (c), and (f), the Department of Health and Human Services (HHS) is recommending that the substance cannabidiol (CBD) and its salts be controlled in Schedule V of the CSA. CBD is a cannabinoid with no significant affinity for cannabinoid receptors (CB, or CB2). It also does not have significant affinity for other sites in the brain, including opioid, GABA, dopamine, norepinephrine, serotonin, glutamate, adenosine, histamine, ion channels, or monoamine transporters. CBD, in a rat drug discrimination study, did not generalize to delta-9-tetrahydrocannabinol (THC), suggesting it does not have cannabinoid-like effects. It also

---

251 *Congress and the FDA May Square Off Over CBD*. By Sean Williams. MOTLEY FOOL. Jan 18, 2020

252 *Bipartisan Group of Representatives Introduces Bill that Would Give FDA Authority to Regulate CBD as a Dietary Supplement.* NATIONAL LAW REVIEW. Thursday, January 16, 2020

does not produce cannabinoid-like responses in the tetrad test with rats. In a separate drug discrimination study, CBD did not generalize to midazolam. CBD is not self-administered by rats, suggesting that it does not have sufficiently rewarding properties to induce reinforcement. In a human abuse potential (HAP) study with CBD, there were slight but statistically significant increases in positive subjective responses after administration of high and supratherapeutic doses of CBD. These responses were just outside the acceptable placebo range, and were much less than those produced by the two positive control drugs: THC and alprazolam. CBD also does not appear to produce physical dependence. CBD as the single active ingredient in a drug product formulation is not yet marketed or available for sale in any country."[253]

In this petition, the department of HHS *proved* all ten criteria required to move a substance to a less restrictive schedule. In the response, the DEA agreed with them, but stated it was not possible to reschedule CBD, due to international agreements:

"Notwithstanding these three findings, there are international scheduling considerations that also impact our final recommendation. Although CBD is not listed in the schedules of the 1961, 1971, or 1988 United Nations International Drug Control Conventions ... Schedule I of the 1961 Convention does include "extracts" of cannabis. In a report published following its November 2017 meeting (Report), the Expert Committee on Drug Dependence of the World Health Organization (ECDD) stated that CBD that is produced as an extract of cannabis is currently included in Schedule I of the 1961 Convention. Subsequently, in the April 6, 2018, DEA Letter, DEA asserted that given the controls mandated by the 1961 Convention, the United States would not be able to keep its obligations under the treaty if CBD were decontrolled under the CSA. The CSA contemplates that scheduling decisions will be made in accordance with treaty obligations. For example, under section 201(d)(I) of the CSA, if control of a substance is required under an international treaty or convention in effect on October 27, 1970, the Attorney General is required to impose controls on such substance by placing it under the schedule he deems most appropriate to carry out such obligations. Here, DEA has requested that HHS conduct a medical and scientific evaluation and provide a scheduling recommendation for CBD. In responding to this request, FDA will not recommend that DEA take action that will cause the United States to be unable to keep its treaty obligations. Thus, if control of CBD is required under

253 *Department of HHS letter.* Posted by HEMP INDUSTRY DAILY

the treaty obligations of the United States, then to continue maintaining such obligations, and reflecting our scientific findings to the extent currently possible, we recommend CBD and its salts, be placed in the least restrictive CSA schedule, Schedule V. If treaty obligations do not require control of CBD, or the international controls on CBD under the 1961 Convention are removed at some future time, the above recommendation for Schedule V under the CSA would need be revisited promptly to address the change in a key predicate underlying such recommendation."

After this, Dr Giroir stated publicly that CBD must remain on Schedule 1, even though it was his personal opinion it should be reclassified as a supplement. He parroted the same reason given by the DEA: CBD cannot be rescheduled, because of international treaties. This "catch-22" in the CSA works to the benefit of the pharmaceutical industry.

President Trump, and his legal team appear more concerned with international treaties, than his promise to stand behind medical cannabis one hundred percent. This is made appearent in the DEA memo. These regulations purport a slavish adherence to international law.

This memo presents this legal opinion as proof of it is constitutional for domestic law to be dependent on foreign treaties:

> "An international agreement has the force of domestic U.S. law if it is self-executing or if Congress has implemented it by legislation. See Medellín v. Texas, 552 U.S. 491, 504–05 (2008). Here, Congress has executed the Single Convention in the CSA."

When the facts of this case are considered, it appears other rulings prove *the opposite*. A foreign national claimed his rights under the Vienna convention were violated:

> "Jose Medellin, a Mexican national, was convicted and sentenced to death for participating in the gang rape and murder of two teenage girls in Houston. Medellin raised a post-conviction challenge arguing that the state had violated his rights under the Vienna Convention, a treaty to which the United States is a party." [254]

This man attempted to escape a conviction in this country, by claiming his rights under an international treaty were violated. This is an inversion to domestic law being dependent on international agreements, as with the CSA. His argument was rejected:

---

254 ***Medellin v. Texas***. OYEZ

"Medellin argued that the Constitution gives the President broad power to ensure that treaties are enforced, and that this power extends to the treatment of treaties in state court proceedings. The Texas Court of Criminal Appeals rejected each of Medellin's arguments and dismissed his petition. The court interpreted Sanchez-Llamas as standing for the principle that rulings of the ICJ are not binding on state courts."

If State *courts* are not bound by international agreements, why must state law follow the CSA, which is dependent on international agreements? It appears the ruling in this case argues *against* their case. International treaties should never be placed above our right to due process under the fifth amendment. This is exactly what the CSA does, a law Trump wholeheartedly supports.

In the response to this petition, we witness the denial of due process—even for the department of HHS. Athough this agency passed all 10 requirements for rescheduling under the law, the petition was still denied due to international treaties. This ruling by the DEA proves due process under the constitution is violated by the CSA. When even a government agency cannot navigate this process with hard evidence, how can the average citizen even have a chance?

Other rulings that establish precedent make the opposite argument—all foreign treaties must be adhered to, *unless* they violate U.S. Law:

"The treaty is . . . a law made by the proper authority, and the courts of justice have no right to annul or disregard any of its provisions, unless they violate the Constitution of the United States." Doe v. Braden, 57 U.S. (16 How.) 635, 656 (1853).

"It need hardly be said that a treaty cannot change the Constitution or be held valid if it be in violation of that instrument." The Cherokee Tobacco, 78 U.S. (11 Wall.), 616, 620 (1871).

The right for a U.S. citizen to have due process is violated if a foreign treaty is the final arbitor. The CSA is a law that can affect life, and liberty, and our rights to challenge this law in court has been taken away. The Attorney General cannot even reschedule CBD, unless international treaties comply.

The lawyers working for Richard Nixon, and the 91st congress had the CSA written so *any* U.S. official—the President, Congress, the Attorney General, or the head of HHS—would violate their oath under the constitution if they reschedule any substance contrary to these international agreements. This is a violation of our fifth amendment rights under the constitution.

Trump Requests Funds to Regulate CBD

The Food and Drug Administration can only test new drugs, or regulate pharmaceuticals or supplements. As stated, many have petitioned the White House to reclassify CBD as a supplement, but to no avail. However, President Trump has requested funds for the FDA to regulate CBD:

> "Trump's proposal asks for an additional $5 million next fiscal year for the U.S. Food and Drug Administration to regulate cannabis and its derivatives, including CBD. The president also asked for more money to oversee hemp farmers.... The FDA last May started reviewing federal regulations for hemp-derived CBD after the 2018 Farm Bill federally legalized hemp and its derivatives. The review has yet to go public. The $5 million boost in Trump's budget would help advance the FDA's regulations for products containing CBD while allowing the agency to enforce the law against making unsubstantiated medical claims about their products, the FDA said in a statement. "FDA is seeing a signicant increase in activity relating to the marketing of unlawful cannabis-derived products, especially those containing cannabidiol, since the Farm Bill passed," the agency noted."[255]

Because the FDA cannot regulate any Schedule 1 substance, and CBD continues to be listed in Schedule 1, these funds cannot be used to regulate this substance as a supplement. However, this agency can use these funds in two ways: implementing fines against businesses that sell it illegally, or to test new drugs based on cannabinoids derived from Hemp.

The new rules for cannabis research approved by the Trump Administration proves this is the plan. It will give billions to the pharmaceutical industry, but only if raw CBD oil remains tightly controlled. It is controlled this way now in the law, but the Trump Administration has not yet enforced these laws. This would not be a smart thing to do, *especially* before reelection.

The new rules for cannabis research (or Hemp research) keep both CBD and THC on Schedule 1, but allow drug companies to profit off of new pharmaceuticals. This shift in resources will give the pharmaceutical industry a "cannabinoid bonanza." This future plan might explain proposed cuts in other agencies:

> "The plan is allocating $35.4 billion for the NIH—estimated to be somewhere between $4.5 and $6 billion less than in the current financial year—and is accompanied by other cuts including a $1 billion reduction for the National Science Foundation (NSF). Among the biggest losers within the NIH are the National Cancer

255 *President Trump requests additional funds to regulate CBD, hemp.* By Laura Drotle. HEMP INDUSTRY DAILY. February 12, 2020

Institute, which would see $900 million carved off its budget to $5.2 billion, and the National Institute of Allergy and Infectious Diseases (NIAID), which would get $4.75 billion, a drop of $750 million, according to a Health and Human Services document (PDF). The move has been attacked by research bodies including the American Association of Immunologists, which says (PDF) that the proposed cut "would devastate important research intended to prevent, treat, and cure innumerable diseases, in part by funding 2,824 fewer research project grants and cutting short the work of many talented and dedicated scientists." Critics are incensed that the cuts to the NIH come alongside a 5% increase in defense spending plus an $8.6 billion request for funding of the Mexican border wall. "Ultimately, the president's proposed $2.7 trillion in spending cuts will leave the nation less healthy and less safe," says Benjamin Corb, public affairs director for the American Society for Biochemistry and Molecular Biology (ASBMB). "While it is important to tackle the federal deficit and balance budgets, the scientific community should not shoulder that burden." To be clear, the Administration's budget proposals have no legal standing and are often torn up by Congress, with plenty of resistance expected this time around with Democrats in command of the House. In the last two years, similar NIH funding cut requests haven't made it through thanks to bipartisan support for the agency, with Congress in fact agreeing to increase the funding made available. Still, the FDA does rather better in Trump's plan, with a total budget of $6.1 billion from October that according to the proposals is a $643 million increase on fiscal 2019. The allocation includes $55 million to support the agency's efforts to curb the opioid epidemic and another $55 million to advance digital healthcare technologies. Advocacy group the Alliance for a Stronger FDA says it is "quite pleased" with the proposed increase in appropriated funding for the regulator, although it puts the increase over the previous year at a smaller figure of $362 million, the net of existing and proposed user fees. Nevertheless, that would help "hire needed scientific personnel to carry out the FDA's far-ranging mission," it adds."[256]

This budget proposal reduces research money for various agencies in the National Institutes of Health (NIH,) including the National Cancer Institute. This shift in resources—combined with the new rules for cannabis research—reveal the reason for this proposed budget. People appointed by the President to key positions have ties to an industry poised to reap a "cannabinoid bonanza."

256 *Trump's budget plan puts squeeze on NIH, boosts FDA* by Phil Taylor. FIERCE BIOTECH Mar 12, 2019

This is only possible if CBD remains an illegal substance, and current law is enforced.

THC More Therapeutic than CBD

According to the plan on cannabis, any research on THC above 0.3% must be approved by the DEA, as it states in the regulations of the CSA. These rules are so costly, and take so much time to navigate, this process has scared many companies away from cannabis research. In these new rules, the only thing that really changes is that pharmaceutical companies will be able to investigate new cannabinoid drugs, derived from Hemp. None of this research be performed THC, *unless the DEA approves*.

Some believe that CBD, and not THC, is the medicinal substance. They think THC is only an intoxicant, but the medicinal properties are found in the other cannabinoids. Many studies prove this belief is not true:

"The marijuana compound CBD, or cannabinol, is surging in popularity in the wellness community, for its alleged health benefits, without the high normally associated with pot. But a new study suggests that marijuana's main active ingredient, THC (tetrahydrocannabinol) — the one that gives users a high — may be more responsible for the plant's therapeutic effects. The researchers looked at data from more than 3,000 people who had tried marijuana to relieve medical symptoms. These participants had all tracked their marijuana use with an app on their smartphones. The study found that higher THC levels were strongly linked with reported symptom relief. In contrast, levels of CBD were not linked with symptom relief. [25 Odd Facts About Marijuana] "Despite the conventional wisdom… that only CBD has medical benefits while THC merely makes one high, our results suggest that THC may be more important than CBD in generating therapeutic benefits," study co-author Jacob Miguel Vigil, associate professor in the Department of Psychology at the University of New Mexico (UNM), said in a statement."[257]

Under Trump's this new plan, drug companies could make a fortune from these new products. Unless the President agrees to reclassify CBD as a supplement, it will continue to be illegal, and there is no reason this a "law and order" President would not instruct government agencies to enforce these laws. After all, it's existence on the shelves is a violation of the international treaties, he has pressured his allies to follow.

------

257 ***THC vs. CBD: Which Marijuana Compound Is More Beneficial?*** By Rachael Rettner. LIVE SCIENCE. February 28, 2019

Pharmaceutical Money, World health, and the European Union

As we have read, the European Union has pushed back their vote on the rescheduling of CBD, and cannabis until December. They have announced they will likely vote to keep CBD on schedule 5 of the 1961 drug treaty, due to "international obligations." Due to the fact President Trump's new "Hemp-cannabis regulatory scheme" is based on a strict redefinition of these treaties, his Administration likely pressured the EU into having this sudden change of heart.

However, it is also possible the pharmaceutical industry has bought off individual members of the EU. The same companies that have corrupted almost every aspect of American government, are international companies, and have also corrupted members of the European Union:

> The study concludes that corruption in the health sector occurs in all EU MSs and that both the nature and the prevalence of corruption typologies differ across the EU member States. The study shows that there is no single policy in the successful fight against corruption in the health sector. What is needed is a combination of effective generic anti-corruption policies and practices (legislation, enforcement), policies and practices aimed at addressing fundamental health system weaknesses (managerial and financial), a general rejection of corruption by society (including a self-regulation by health sector actors), and specific anti-corruption in healthcare policies and practices."[258]

Consider how ridiculous, and unfair the drug laws of the United States are. Consider the schemes of the most intelligent con-men, and compare them to the Controlled Substance Act. No substance can be placed into a different Schedule of the CSA unless the majority of *every nation on earth* votes to reschedule it. Nixon helped create a law that "locks in stone" these laws perpetually, and make any change almost impossible.

It is inconceivable that pharmaceutical money did not somehow influence the regulations of the CSA. It works in their favor. Since they are giving money to every elected official, including Donald Trump, it makes since someone was bribed, to craft this deceiving law. People who have likely passed away.

Pharmaceutical money has also corrupted the World Health Organization:

> "Serious questions have been raised about whether the World Health Organization is using patient groups as a conduit for receiving proscribed donations from the pharmaceutical industry. Email correspondence passed to the BMJ seems to show that

---

258 **Study on Corruption in the Healthcare Sector.** October 2013

in June 2006 Benedetto Saraceno, the director of WHO's
department of mental health and substance abuse, suggested
that a patient organisation accept $10 000 (£5000; €7000) from
GlaxoSmithKline (GSK) on WHO's behalf. The sum was then to be
passed on to WHO—ostensibly with the intention of obscuring
the origins of the donation. GSK withdrew its offer of funding
when it learnt that acceptance was conditional on obscuring its
origin. However, the email exchange indicates that other sums of
money originating from drug companies may have already been
channelled to WHO through patient groups." [259]

Pharmaceutical companies have corrupted almost every aspect of
government—no matter *which* government you are talking about. Every year,
politicians receive millions of these funds, many times after they leave office. Of
course, you cannot blame them for taking money. But you can blame them for
turning their backs on the sick for this money.

Many people are against cannabis, and CBD legalization for only *one*
reason—they have been bought off. And it is not out of imagination that a
man who has almost *2 billion dollars* might have a plan to double that money,
sometime after he leaves office. *"The rich get richer..."*

259 *Who's funding WHO?* THE BMJ. PUBMED. February 17, 2007

CHAPTER 10:
VOTE AGAINST THE "SWAMP" OF GOVERNMENT CANNABIS PROHIBITION

Big Money, and legal trickery is being used against the legalization of cannabis. The drug laws written by the lawyers of Richard Nixon, the 91st Congress carefully craft this deception, that attempts to satisfy the Constitutional requirement for due process with regulations impossible for even the department of HHS to successfully navigate. Even this agency could not have CBD rescheduled because it violates international agreements. Nixon's "catch-22" in the Controlled Substance Act cannot be broken.

And, the legal team of Donald Trump has interpreted these regulations even stricter. His lawyers released the legal memo instructing the DEA to change it's policies, regulate cannabis as opium, seize all crops after harvest, and establish a government monopoly—because international agreements require it. As far as drug laws are concerned, Trump whole-heartedly embraces the "swamp" of the United Nations.

President Trump assembled *the Marijuana Policy Coordination Committee*, and has given one quarter of his yearly salary towards an anti-cannabis warning posted by the Surgeon General, full of errors. The appointment of former CEO's, and lobbyists from the pharmaceutical industry makes his anti-cannabis actions even more suspicious.

In any case, despite recent reforms at the state level, strong opposition continues to exist, both in the laws Trump refuses to change, and financially. *The facts do not add-up to the promises of Donald Trump about cannabis.*

Publicly Supported Corey Gardner

After Attorney General Jeff Sessions rescinded the Cole Memo, Senator Corey Gardner held up President Trump's nominations in the Senate. After this, the President made assurances to the Senator that he would not target the legal cannabis industry[260]. After this phone call, Senator Gardner introduced a bill to reform cannabis laws, and the President was asked about his support:

> "A bill that would protect state marijuana laws from federal interference received a major plug on Friday when President Donald Trump said he probably would back the measure, introduced a day earlier by two U.S. senators. "(I) probably will end up supporting" it, Trump told reporters during a 20-minute exchange with reporters at the White House, according to pool reports."[261]

This soundbite of the President was spread throughout the media, and has influenced voters. But consider the context of this promise. *After* the President had *privately* established an anti-cannabis cabinet, and *after* the President *privately* circulated the memo inside the DEA, he publicly promised to support the Senators cannabis reforms.

President Trump lied to Senator Gardner, and the American voters at the same time. It is not possible to support cannabis reforms, and believe the DEA must seize the entire cannabis crop to comply with international treaties. The Memo was released to the DEA on June 6, 2018. One day later, Trump made these promises to Senator Gardner.

The same is true with Trump's promise about honoring states rights on this issue:

> "President Donald Trump reiterated Friday that his administration
> is allowing states to set their own marijuana policies. At a press
> briefing Friday, the president was asked by DC Examiner reporter
> Steven Nelson whether cannabis would be federally legalized

---

260 "U.S. Sen. Cory Gardner on Friday formally ended a three-month standoff with the Justice Department over federal marijuana law enforcement, saying he received assurances from President Donald Trump that the agency wouldn't interfere with Colorado's marijuana industry. In an announcement met with caution by industry observers, Gardner said he wouldn't block any more Senate-confirmable Justice nominees. He undertook that protest after a controversial January decision by U.S. Attorney General Jeff Sessions to void an Obama-era policy that generally left alone states that had legalized the drug. Trump's pledge came during a long phone conversation Wednesday night, Gardner said." *President Trump to Cory Gardner: Colorado's legal marijuana won't be targeted by Jeff Sessions, Justice Department* By MARK K. MATTHEWS and ALICIA WALLACE The Denver Post PUBLISHED: April 13, 2018

261 *Donald Trump would "probably" support legalizing Colorado's marijuana industry — through bid by Cory Gardner and Elizabeth Warren* By Mark Matthews. THE DENVER POST .June 8, 2018

while he was in office. The comments come one day after the surgeon general issued a warning against the use of cannabis by adolescents and pregnant women."[262]

President Trump reiterated public support for cannabis reforms, only *one day* after the Surgeon General posted the refutable warnings about cannabis he financed. The two are at odds, as publicly supporting Senator Gardner's reforms after all his actions against cannabis.

Vice President Biden, Kamala Harris, and Cannabis

President Trump will take any issue, and use it for his benefit. Consider the charges he has made against Joe Biden, and Kamala Harris about their positions on cannabis, in light of all of the information in this book. He has criticized Joe Biden for passing laws that incarcerated minorities for cannabis use:

> "Joe Biden's policies destroyed millions of black lives" due to his role in advancing anti-drug laws and other criminal justice policies, it states. "Joe Biden may not remember. But we do."[263]

This is the "pot calling the kettle black." President Trump supports keeping cannabis on Schedule 1, tired to nominate a drug Czar that wants to lock up drug users in a "Hospital/prison," and gladly supports current laws that allow states to craft their own policies, and imprison cannabis users. Minorities disproportionately have their lives ruined by these laws.

When all of the actions of the President against cannabis are considered, these claims against the other candidates become laughable. He also has slammed Kamala Harris for prosecuting over a thousand people for cannabis:

> "California Sen. Kamala Harris is officially Joe Biden's running mate, making her the first Black and South Asian American woman to make a major party's presidential ticket. The announcement was made yesterday, and the selection has already drawn criticism from notable GOP members, including President Donald Trump, who targeted Harris's cannabis history. Trump first called Harris "nastier than Pocahontas," a dig at his rival Sen. Elizabeth Warren, who has claimed Cherokee Native American ancestry in the past. The President later labeled Harris "the meanest, most horrible, most disrespectful of anybody in the U.S. Senate."..."I think as attorney general in California, the position that Kamala Harris

---

262 ***President Trump reiterates his administration will let states legalize marijuana.*** MARIJUANA MOMENT. September 3, 2019

263 ***Trump Reelection Campaign Attacks Biden As 'Architect' Of The War On Drugs.***By Kyle Yaeger. June 20, 2020.

has held much longer than she's been a United States senator, people will dig into that record," she told Fox. "It looks like she left nobody happy." "She is seen by those on the far left, many speaking up last night, as not sufficiently for criminal justice reform," Conway added. "She locked up over 1,500 people or so on marijuana charges, and by others who are for public safety and law and order, she is seen as somebody who is soft on some of those criminals. And so, I think she has a very mixed record there that people will dig into."[264]

These charges are true, but for Trump's campaign to make them is extremely hypocritical. President Trump has a gall trying to get the upper hand on this issue. However, honesty is always the best policy, and consistency speaks truth. The pharmaceutical industry donates large sums of money to *both political* parties. Joe Biden has also received donations from pharmaceutical companies:

> "...Trump might not be alone in trusting unqualified pharmaceutical executives with policy decisions. The Revolving Door Project has found 2020 candidates Joe Biden and Pete Buttigieg are both accepting significant donations from the pharmaceutical industry. The rallying of donations around these two candidates indicates the industry is already placing bets to install its allies in key positions across the next administration and minimize government oversight on, say, lowering drug prices." [265]

Take note, this article admits that the pharmaceutical industry:

> "...is already placing bets to install its allies in key positions..."

The fight on our hands is clear. A vote this election towards cannabis reforms this year could end years of prohibition, or set back reforms another decade. The "web" of the drug companies can only be broken if laws are passed that make donations from *any* company, or union illegal. This is the kind of prohibition we really need—on political influence, not cannabis.

When considering this issue, three factors should be considered (1) The length of time the people have struggled to correct this bad law; (2) The potential influence political parties have on their candidates (3) "Lame Duck" status—the fear of reelection taken away.

We have fought against prohibition for a long time. The federal

264 *Trump and GOP Already Attacking Kamala Harris over Marijuana Record*. By Brendan Bures. August 13, 2020

265 *Biden and Buttigieg See Pharma Money as the Cure For Campaign Woes*. By Andrea Beaty. March 1, 2020

government under Donald Trump has worked against any reforms. *After almost one hundred years*, laws are finally being reformed at the state level. If the documents quoted in this book prove the President's true intentions, it is possible *one* election could reverse reforms that have taken twenty years.

Thousands of people would suddenly be denied the ability to treat their illness with a substance safer than the majority of prescription medications. Some would argue with this statement, but substances that kill, are substances that kill—and cannabis is not one of them.

The influence of political parties on their leaders should be considered, if you are voting to put an end to these insane laws once and for all. Mitch McConnell has stated flatly he doesn't plan to allow a vote on the legalization of cannabis. So, we know where the leadership of the Republican Party stands on this issue. The Democrat Party has stated that they will legalize cannabis, *despite* Joe Biden's position on this issue:

> "In a news interview July 11, U.S. Senator Edward Markey (D-MA) said a Democratic Congress will legalize marijuana in 2021 despite opposition from the party's presumptive presidential nominee, Joe Biden. Sen. Markey stated: "We'll have the majority of the votes in the United States Senate. And I know [Senate Minority Leader Chuck Schumer (D-NY)] has moved in that direction, he'll be the majority leader in January. I think we'll have votes to just move it, and the science has moved there." Biden remains opposed to adult-use legalization, but Markey insists that supporters will have the votes to pass it anyway. He went on to say: "From my perspective, this is another issue that's just right there on the ballot in November. We'll move very quickly in January to change these laws to make sure that there are national protections which are put in place." [266]

Democrats in the House promise to advance a bill to legalize cannabis, regardless of Joe Biden's position. That is why the possible "lame duck" status of Donald Trump should also be a deciding factor in this election. Whether you believe it or not, Donald Trump is restraining himself right now. That's right. Every President running for reelection does this. They "hold back," on certain issues, out of fear of losing voters. *How much* depends on the honesty of the candidate. They are almost all dishonest; but there are *degrees* to dishonesty.

President Trump has claimed "executive privilege" many times over key documents related to cannabis reforms, or lack of reforms. Why? He doesn't want the voters to know. We still do not know the content of the written reports submitted by the *Marijuana Policy Coordination Committee.*

Unlike Joe Biden, Donald Trump has a strong, abrasive will. He will do whatever he wants, and has—many times by executive order. Ruling like this

---

266 *Pot Prohibition's Days Are Numbered By John Persinos.* INVESTING DAILY July 14, 2020

could be unconstitutional, depending on the action. This "strong will" approach of the President will likely raise it's ugly head towards legal cannabis after reelection. Already, cannabis prohibition has hurt many people, *but it could get worse*.

Cannabis Prohibition Denies Transplants

Before President Trump, and his advisors use federal laws against cannabis legalization, they should consider the ramifications of their actions. Because of federal regulations, people are routinely denied organ transplants for cannabis use:

> "A Utah man who initially was denied a life-saving lung transplant because marijuana was found in his system died over the weekend. After being admitted to the University of Utah in December, Hancey, of Park City, was put on life support two weeks later and was denied a transplant earlier this month after traces of THC — the main ingredient in pot — were found in his system. ...Mark Hancey said his son smoked pot with his friends on Thanksgiving after being drug-free for a year. "It's not like he's a smoker for 30 years and [had] deteriorating lungs because of that," Mark Hancey told KSL.com. But the hospital, according to its policy, does not transplant organs in patients with "active alcohol, tobacco, or illicit drug use or dependencies," spokeswoman Kathy Wilets said at the time, adding that the policy is intended to give patients a higher chance of surviving surgery and completing their recovery process."[267]

Before organ transplantation, a drug test is performed, and the recipient is usually denied if THC is found in their system. This is the normal "hospital policy," based on decisions made at the *Organ Procurement and Transplantation Network*, run by the Department of Health, and Human Services (HHS.) Their regulations deny cannabis users organ transplants.

This is another way current federal laws against cannabis are killing people. These are laws the President supports because of "international agreements." If someone dies of organ failure in this country, the United Nations will not care. And if President Trump doesn't *keep his word*, and support cannabis reforms—he is either uninformed, or he also doesn't care.

Oregon lawmakers have introduced a bill to prevent this travesty:

> "Oregon lawmakers may tighten restrictions on the state's organ transplant centers to ensure they don't discriminate against patients based on marijuana use. House Bill 2687, sponsored by

---

267 *Man who was denied lung transplant over marijuana use dies*. By Joshua Rhett Miller April 24, 2017

Rep. Rob Nosse, D-Portland, would stop medical providers from recommending that transplant candidates be removed from the organ waiting list managed by the nonprofit United Network for Organ Sharing because they tested positive for pot, the Statesman Journal reported."[268]

Even people who have had a physician approve the use of medical cannabis can be denied transplants under Federal rules. Routine prescription drugs given to prevent transplant rejection have one bad side effect—cancer[269]. These drugs are the *only option* because of federal laws, which the Trump Administration has more strictly reinterpreted.

And this federal law is likely preventing people from having a *greater chance of success* in transplantation. In animal studies, THC has both anti-cancer, and immunomodulator effects. Scientists believe it can *aid* in transplantation:

"Cannabinoids have emerged as powerful drug candidates for the treatment of inflammatory and autoimmune diseases due to their immunosuppressive properties. While significant clinical and experimental data on the use of cannabinoids as anti-inflammatory agents exist in many autoimmune disease settings, virtually no studies have been performed on their potential role in transplant rejection. Here we suggest a theoretical role for the use of cannabinoids in preventing allograft rejection. While the psychotropic properties of CB1 agonists limit their clinical use, CB2 agonists may offer a new avenue to selectively target immune cells involved in allograft rejection. Moreover, development of mixed CB1/CB2 agonists that cannot cross the blood-brain barrier may help prevent their undesired psychotropic properties. In addition, manipulation of endocannabinoids in vivo by activating their biosynthesis and inhibiting cellular uptake and metabolism may offer yet another pathway to regulate immune response during allograft rejection." (Do Cannabinoids have a therapeutic role in transplantation? TRENDS IN PHARMACOLOGICAL SCIENCE. August 31, 2010[270])

The government is denying people transplants for using a drug that likely *aids* in transplantation, and does not cause cancer, as other drugs used to prevent transplant rejection. The government has it backwards, and these regulations cause hospitals all across the country to make extremely bad decisions. When you go to the polls this November, remember these transplant

---

268 *Bill would aid marijuana users who need organ transplants*. By Jonathan Bach. AP NEWS. February 4, 2019
269 *Immunomodulators and Their Side Effects* AMERICAN CANCER SOCIETY.
270 *Do Cannabinoids have a therapeutic role in transplantation?* TRENDS IN PHARMACOLOGICAL SCIENCES. August 1, 2011

patients, and vote *for* cannabis legalization—and the candidates most likely to support it.

Harsh Prison Sentences

A vote to continue current federal laws against cannabis allow state governments to impose harsh prison sentences, for possessing only a small amount of this plant. Despite a few instances when President Trump has pardoned some of these drug offenders, they were serving decades in jail, and were brought to the attention of the President by friends, or acquaintances.

Hundreds of people everyday are having their lives ruined by harsh state laws. Trump's position of "leaving it up to the states" *sounds* good, but it also leaves it up to the states to ruin lives. One medical marijuana patient had his home raided in Kansas over one plant:

"Larry Burgess has no criminal record. He's a cancer survivor who suffers from seizure disorder. He tried prescription drugs. A cocktail of 23 pills a day didn't cut it. "No seizure medication helped. In fact, my seizures got progressively worse over time. It was terrible. Terrible. At my lowest I contemplated suicide," Burgess said...He faces four criminal charges following a raid near Fredonia, Kansas, which happened more than two years ago. Burgess says it was tough to conceal what worked in a small town. For years, he was almost a shut-in because seizures were so bad and could strike at any moment. He practically disappeared from the community and then was back. "And then I'm able to go back to church. You know, when you're not in church for four years at a time and then you're able to go back to church. I mean, it's just, it's not rocket science," Burgess said. Police crime scene photos show Burgess also posted about his plant on Instagram and how he was doing much better. It's obvious from police body camera video, Burgess was stunned his home was raided over one pot plant."[271]

Although the prosecutor has now dropped some of these charges, it is still unacceptable to serve months in prison for growing one plant to treat an illness. In four years, President Trump has not moved to change any of these laws, instead he uses UN treaties to excuse their existence—and *strengthen them*.

Killed for Legally Possessing both Cannabis and Guns

Police raids have occurred throughout this country in legal cannabis states when someone owns a gun, and a medical cannabis card at the same time. For this reason, if you are a gun owner in a state that allows recreational

---

271 ***Kansas man faces decades in prison for medical marijuana*** Angie Ricono KCTV-5. Feb 12, 2020

cannabis, you should forego obtaining your medical card if you want to own a gun.

Recently, in Potomac, Maryland, police raided a home, and shot a medical cannabis patient while he slept next to his wife in bed:

> "The constitution is dead" was the last tweet ever sent by 21-year-old Duncan Socrates Lemp. On Thursday morning at 4:30 a.m., a Montgomery County SWAT team killed Lemp during a violent attack on his family's home in the affluent Washington suburb of Potomac, Maryland...Why did the SWAT team attack the home as Lemp was sleeping? The initial county police press release referred only to "firearms offenses." County police spokeswoman Mary Davison refused to disclose either the details of Lemp's alleged offense or the affidavit used to justify the raid. Instead, she notified me that my press inquiries were being handled under the Maryland Public Information Act which entitles government agencies to delay responding for weeks or months...Why was Lemp targeted? Lawyer Sandler said that the search warrant referred to Lemp as a "prohibited person" —meaning that he was prohibited from owning firearms. That could mean simply that he had a permit to use medical marijuana —a violation that would apply to tens of thousands of Maryland gun owners who use marijuana despite federal law prohibiting gun ownership combined with pot smoking. A check of Montgomery County court records revealed one offense for Lemp: a speeding ticket from last year. Court records state that Lemp was only 5' 8" and 145 pounds but he was towering enough to terrify a SWAT team into opening fire without warning.[272]

These police, and the prosecutors who approved this raid hard-headily use federal drug laws to violate due process, and murder.

Alcohol impairs more; It is more dangerous to use booze around firearms than cannabis. But this doesn't matter, if something is a "prohibited substance" according to federal law. It is an "illegal drug," and the police treat it's use around guns like they are facing the mob. Instead, a man was killed for treating his illness with a plant.

The State of Pennsylvania warns that despite the legality of medical cannabis, it is illegal under federal law to own both cannabis and a gun:

> It is legal under Pennsylvania law for the holder of a validly issued patient Medical Marijuana Card to possess approved forms of medical marijuana. However, as per the United States

272 *Did Maryland Police Shoot and Kill a Sleeping Man?* By Jim Bovard. AMERICAN CONSERVATIVE. March 14, 2020

Department of Justice, Bureau of Alcohol, Tobacco, Firearms and Explosives (BATFE), the possession of medical marijuana remains a violation of federal law, and possession of a valid Medical Marijuana Card and/or the use of medical marijuana makes you an "unlawful user of or addicted to any controlled substance" who is prohibited by federal law from the purchase or acquisition, possession, or control of a firearm pursuant to 18 U.S.C. § 922(g)(3), and 27 C.F.R. § 478.32(a)(3). The BATFE's position is set forth in its September 21, 2011, Open Letter to all Federal Firearms Licensees, which states in part that "[t]herefore, any person who uses or is addicted to marijuana, regardless of whether his or her State has passed legislation authorizing marijuana use for medicinal purposes, is an unlawful user of or addicted to a controlled substance, and is prohibited by Federal law from possessing firearms or ammunition."... Likewise, the mere possession of a Medical Marijuana Card will give rise to an inference that you are an "unlawful user of or addicted to" a controlled substance, pursuant to 27 C.F.R. § 478.11."[273]

A medical cannabis patient is not an "addicted user," anymore than a hypertensive patient is addicted to blood pressure medication. People who have a serious medical condition should not be judged this way. How many people thought that their votes counted when voting for medical cannabis, only to be arrested for possessing a "prohibited substance" with firearms? President Trump supports these bad federal laws. If you are a medical cannabis user, he doesn't support your second amendment rights—or at least not enough to change these laws.

Children taken from Parents

The atrocity of federal prohibition against cannabis empowers the Department of Social Services to take children away from their parents. Good parents with a serious medical condition—such as epilepsy—should not have their homes broken up for saving their own lives. If parents *die* from epilepsy, their children will be without them *forever*. In one instance, social services took a child away from her mother for cannabis use, and that child was abused, and later killed by the foster mother:

> "2-year-old taken away from parents because they used marijuana, killed by foster mother. Alex Hill was placed in foster care after her father admitted to using marijuana according to the Houston Press. Joshua Hill told Texas child welfare investigators that he smoked after the child was in bed at night. A case worker determined that the father's marijuana use and the mother's

---

273 *Firearms Information*. PENN STATE POLICE

medical condition (frequent seizures) warranted removal from the home. The toddler had appeared healthy and happy with her parents, but she was placed into the foster care system in early 2013. On Tuesday Alex's foster mother, Sherill Small, was sentenced to life in prison for the July 2013 death of the little girl, who would have turned four on Friday. "[274]

President Trump supports federal laws that allow this to happen. Even if the foster parents do not kill the child, these children will by emotionally scarred. The government has it's priories backwards. Cannabis users are like anyone else; they can be good or bad parents. Donald Trump *in the least* supports the status quo that has allowed this to happen. But considering his actions, it is likely he will restrict all access to cannabis at a future time.

The Effect on Drug Testing

Throughout history, a segment of the population has always sought some form of intoxication. Anyone who thinks they can change this by the "letter of the law" doesn't understand human nature. The question every society must honesty answer is, what substance is more dangerous? Alcohol kills. Cannabis does not.

Some people, like diabetics, cannot use alcohol. Alcohol turns into sugar, and could cause the loss of limbs, or even kill them. Additionally, many companies drug test for cannabis, because it is illegal. This causes many people to use this more dangerous substance. Alcohol leads to violence, and numerous health problems.

Cannabis use is drug tested because of prohibition. This makes it's use problematic. THC is stored in the fat cells, and shows up in a drug test *for up to 30 days*. This fact, combined with drug testing, indirectly puts people at risk. Not only do some use alcohol as a replacement, the stimulant class of drugs leave the body quickly. In about two to four days, drugs like methamphetamine, adderall, and ecstasy no longer show up in a drug test. Some people are using these drugs, or alcohol, instead of cannabis because they fear losing their jobs.

For instance, a truck driver could begin a three day journey, use one of these drugs at the beginning of his trip, and it would likely be out of his system by the time he reached his destination, and could be drug tested. Cannabis use after work would be safer—both for the individual, and society.

Physicians Are Not Properly Trained

Cannabis prohibition is detrimental to the education of our physicians. One of the main systems of the human body is the endocannabinoid system, named after cannabis:

---

274 *2-year-old taken away from parents because they used marijuana, killed by foster mother*. FOX43. November 6, 2014

"The endogenous cannabinoid system—named for the plant that led to its discovery—is one of the most important physiologic systems involved in establishing and maintaining human health. Endocannabinoids and their receptors are found throughout the body: in the brain, organs, connective tissues, glands, and immune cells. With its complex actions in our immune system, nervous system, and virtually all of the body's organs, the endocannabinoids are literally a bridge between body and mind. By understanding this system, we begin to see a mechanism that could connect brain activity and states of physical health and disease."[275]

Many physicians are unaware this vital signaling system of the human body exists, because only 13% of medical schools teach it in their curriculum:

"The lack of education from grade school through grad school and medical school regarding cannabis, cannabinoids and the endocannabinoid system (ECS) is directly a result of bad policy. Up and down this is due to the government dealing with many psychoactive substances on a criminal justice basis not as medicine and not following the science. Much of education problem can be traced to our medical schools. The majority of US medical schools are not even addressing the ECS, arguably the largest neurotransmitter system in the human brain, let alone the medicinal utility of cannabis and the appropriate cannabis dosage for various medical indications. In 2013, Cardiologist Dr. David Allen did a preliminary survey to determine which schools teach the ECS and found that only a total of 13 percent of U.S. medical schools even mentioned it. "[276]

There are several possible reasons for this ignorance. Some colleges could be pressured to leave this out of the curriculum by pharmaceutical companies after receiving donations; government obstruction due to prohibition; or simple ignorance. It could be a combination of these factors. In any case, we want our physicians to be taught all of the facts.

Relocation Because of Federal Law

All across this country, people have moved from their homes to access medical cannabis. This should not happen in America, which should be a free country. These people should not be forced to have their lives uprooted,

---

275 *Getting High on the Endocannabinoid System*. By Bradley E Alger, Ph.D. CEREBUM. November-December 2013
276 *The Systemic Lack of Education About the Endocannabinoid System Leads to Widespread Ignorance About Cannabis* February 10, 2019 by David Bearman, M.D. (reprinted)

because people in our government slavishly support international drug treaties over individual rights. Colorado was one of the first states that witnessed this emigration:

> "She's been on strict diets. She's had brain surgery. Nothing reduced the 15 or so seizures she had every day since she was 5 months old that kept her from walking steadily, feeding herself or talking. Her parents, Maria and Mark, had run out of options. Then they heard about a strain of marijuana grown in Colorado that reduced the number of seizures in children with severe epilepsy. "We really tried everything with Greta," says Maria Botker, a nurse. "We put our child through brain surgery, so a plant like marijuana was not going to scare me." In November, Maria and Greta headed west to find a miracle. Mark and the couple's two other daughters, 13 and 10, stayed on the family's farm in Minnesota. Maria and Greta joined a migration of parents who, after trying countless methods to ease their children's crippling seizures, are packing up their families and moving to Colorado. The state has become a refuge for those families for two reasons: Colorado has the most liberal laws for use of marijuana, and it has opened a market for a strain called Charlotte's Web that is believed to be effective for people with severe epilepsy."[277]

Simply "supporting states rights" on this issue is not enough—and Trump's actions indicate even this isn't true. Remember, he said that he was only allowing states to make that decision *"now."* But some states make criminals of their citizens for accessing a natural medication. So people take the expensive, but necessary step of relocation. They move to save their lives, or the lives of their children.

If President Trump shuts down the cannabis industry, the sacrifices of all these sick people will be in vain. This should be unacceptable. No state or government should be able to prohibit people from possessing any plant, or natural substance—unless it *kills*, or has proven to be more dangerous than any prescription medication. By default, the FDA should regulate plants as supplements. Only if these plants intoxicate, should the government be allowed to regulate them as alcohol. But prohibition by default, until a substance is proven safe, is backwards.

Certainly, governments should be allowed to make laws regulating, or prohibiting refined, or synthetic substances. Drugs such as heroin or cocaine are refined. Synthetic drugs are usually new substances. Plants, and other natural substances were created by God. Governments should not overreach their power, by outlawing what God has created.

------

277 ***Parents move to Colorado for 'miracle' pot for children*** Marisol Bello USA TODAY February 17, 2014

This short-sighted "zero tolerance" attitude has harmed millions of lives. For instance, coca tea in it's raw form is not psychoactive, and does not create a "high." It is not the same as cocaine, but similar to a strong cup of coffee. Opening the coca tea market would take billions of dollars away from the drug cartels, and help raise millions of lives out of poverty. Violence would be reduced because of both factors. The effect the legalization of cannabis has had on state governments improving their economies would be a microcosm of a legal coca tea market. There would be no need for emigrating to America for economic opportunities. There would be no discussion about Trump's "wall."

Of course, import laws could prevent this plant from being brought into the country in bulk, causing possible diversion into cocaine production. Import laws could be designed so it could must be prepackaged where it is grown, and sold as tea. Cocaine manufacturing would become economically unprofitable if this were to occur. This would cause a great change in that region. But we cant do this, because it is a violation of international treaties. Because of international laws, we are forced to continuing financing the drug cartels of Central, and South America.

In 1961, Brazil voted against the inclusion of the coca plant in the 1961 Single Convention on Narcotic Drugs, but the United States objected. A "zero tolerance" position was taken. So, what happened? Instead of having a viable crop to grow, and sell legally throughout the world,[278] drug cartels got rich, while the people in their countries starved.

The led to wars, deaths, cocaine addiction, and a huge immigration problem in the United States. The legalization of one plant not much stronger than coffee could have changed things for the better.

Trump Marijuana Promise At Center Of Feud

In Tweets, Mark Meadows, the White House Chief of Staff denied that President Trump made any promises to Corey Gardner about cannabis reforms—despite Trump publicly supporting the Senator's bill. In these tweets, Mr Meadows claimed the Senator was misleading voters. When asked about this later, Mr Meadows laughed about the President's cannabis support:

> "President Donald Trump's stance on marijuana legalization became the jumping off point for a spat between a top White House aide, Republican operatives and a reporter on Thursday after Chief of Staff Mark Meadows laughed off a question about the prospects of broad cannabis reform advancing before the election in November. But the controversy wasn't solely about the administration's position on legalization; rather the dispute centered on how freelance reporter Matt Laslo characterized the conversation on Twitter, where he said that Meadows suggested pro-cannabis reform Sen. Cory Gardner (R-CO) "has been

---

278 It is legal in Colombia, Peru, Bolivia, Argentina, and Ecuador

misleading voters on marijuana" and that "Trump has no plan to lift a finger on cannabis legalization or even normalization." The exchange: Laslo: Has there been any talk about moving marijuana legalization ahead of November? Meadows: [Laughs] Laslo: Trump promised it to Gardner. Meadows: [Laughs] Laslo: Some people say that disproportionately it affects minority communities. Meadows: I'm not aware of anything on the agenda for the Senate or the House that would move a bill in that regard. We—the White House has not weighed in on that."[279]

The laugher of Mr. Meadows reveals where the President stands this issue, especially after other news reports—Trump assembled an anti-cannabis cabinet, circulated the Memo within the DEA, that tightened regulations. The President was working against the industry in a number of ways at the time he publicly supported these reforms. Mr Meadows tweets simply reveal the President's true intentions on this issue.

List of Trump's Major Anti-Cannabis Actions

This book reveals many of the "anti-cannabis" actions" of Donald Trump. *Since he took office four years ago, the President has:*

• Assembled an "anti-cannabis cabinet" almost as soon as he took office
• Circulated a memo in the DEA that stated a monopoly must be established, in order to keep international agreements. This memo was the basis for the postponement of a promised plan to accept applications to grow research grade cannabis.
• Attempted to prevent Israel from exporting medical cannabis
• Had the Attorney General end the Cole memorandum, which protected legal cannabis businesses from federal interference.
• Had Canadian cannabis investors banned *for life* from entering the United States due to cannabis investments.
• Refused immigrants entrance into this country who used cannabis, because they were "immoral"
• Denied mental health funds to schools who allowed medical cannabis to be given to sick children
• Gave $100,000 of his salary towards an anti-cannabis campaign based on selected, refutable studies.
• Has has not rebuked, or commented about several members of his Administration, claiming it is his position to keep cannabis illegal
• Denied the use of medical cannabis, and CBD to military vets

---

279 *Alleged Trump Marijuana Promise At Center Of Feud Between White House Aide, Reporter And GOP Operatives.* MEDICAL HEMP NEWS. June 19, 2020

All of these actions paint a picture of a man with an agenda. Despite the shortcomings of Vice President Biden on this issue, the memo Trump circulated inside the Drug Enforcement Agency reveals the future if he is reelected. Cannabis must be regulated as opium, and all crops must be seized by the feds after harvest, to keep UN laws. All state cannabis laws are illegal, according to the words of this memo. That is what President Trump *really* supports, not his thirty second sound bites about this issue.

Pandemic Relief tied to Cannabis Banking Reform

If there is any doubt that this Administration is against any cannabis reforms, consider the second coronavirus stimulus package. Vice President Pence said it is being held up because the Democrats want cannabis banking reforms in the bill:

> "...the bill Pence is complaining about makes it possible for cannabis businesses to safely engage in banking in states where cannabis is legal, which helps those "working-class families" who rely on the cannabis industry. Second, the bill he's referring to will actually save taxpayers money, unlike much of the rest of this relief legislation. The "Secure and Fair Enforcement Act of 2019," a.k.a. the "SAFE Banking Act," would allow legally operating cannabis businesses to have the same legal access to banks, loans, and deposit protections as other legal businesses. Because the sale and possession of marijuana are still forbidden by federal law, banks are reluctant to have any dealings with dispensaries and growers, even when they're legally operating within their home states. This is not a pork-barrel bill. While the marijuana industry would love to have access to federal coronavirus relief, the SAFE Banking Act would allow them only to use banking services the way other businesses do. According to the Congressional Budget Office, passing the bill would actually reduce the federal deficit by $2-3 million dollars a year. This is small potatoes in the grand scheme of things (the federal deficit for 2020 stands so far at $2.8 trillion), but as Reason Foundation Policy Analyst Jacob James Rich observes, legal banking creates a framework for the expansion of the cannabis industry and also improves bookkeeping and revenue and income reporting."[280]

This rider in the bill did *not* give pandemic assistance to cannabis dispensaries—although relief was given to liquor companies in the previous bill. This rider merely allowed a legal business to use the banks. Right now, the

---

280 ***Mike Pence Comes Out Against Marijuana Banking Bill That Would Actually Save Taxpayers Money.*** By Scott Shackford. REASON. August 13, 2020

majority of cannabis dispensaries use cash, and this makes it unsafe—especially since crime has skyrocketed in several cities. The Trump Administration refused to support this measure—even to the point they are willing to deny your pandemic assistance.

This Administration would only take this drastic measure if they were against the legal cannabis market 100%. This banking amendment contains many of the reforms that were in Senator Gardner's bill, which President Trump *claimed* he supported. Instead, he has blocked these reforms, and banks will continue to refuse business from both the legal cannabis industry, or the CBD industry. These banks are afraid of the federal government.

I personally was denied by right to use a payment processor, because I wrote *books* about the medicinal properties of CBD. These were digital downloads designed to help people. The payment processor *Stripe* informed me it was denying my business because I sold CBD. I told them that I did not sell CBD, but I sold *books* about CBD. This was their response:

Hello there,

Thanks for getting back to us.

While I really appreciate you providing us with that clarification, I'm afraid that our existing Restricted Businesses List does not currently allow us to support any businesses that are related to the marijuana industry — this includes businesses and organizations that are not directly selling marijuana or CBD, and are instead providing information and resources to individuals who may be using marijuana.

I'm truly sorry that we cannot do better for you right now. I wish you the very best in everything moving forward, and hope that you're able to find a payment processor better suited to your business. If you have any other questions please let me know and I'll get back to you as soon as possible.

All the best,
Declan

I was not allowed to present valuable information, because this company is afraid of federal laws. CBD can save an epileptic child's life, but that information cannot be published according to the business rules of Stripe. A business should not deny the free expression of the first amendment because *the government disapproves*.

Through pressure, the feds can selectively curtail important information, *as Stripe does*. According the regulations of Stripe, PUBMED could not use them to republish hundreds of pre-clinical studies from their site about cannabis. You have read this book. Have I given any instructions about how to use cannabis? No. Neither have I in any of my other books. But even if this were the case, free speech, and free expression of truth should never be selectively curtailed.

The Vice President is against these banking reforms, and has also received contributions from pharmaceutical companies:

> Amid speculation that Pence could mount his own presidential bid—or replace Trump if he leaves office early — the former Indiana governor and U.S. congressman has been directly lobbied by major health care and drug companies, Wall Street firms, oil and gas interests and industry groups interested in shaping a federal infrastructure privatization initiative. Pence's office has also been lobbied by his former congressional chief of staff on behalf of insurance, defense contracting and telecommunications companies — and that lobbying revolved around health care policy, defense spending and net neutrality. Pence has enthusiastically backed the policies by the lobbying firms."[281]

Many of the same companies that have given large sums of money against cannabis reforms also gave to the Mike Pence. This in, and of itself does not indicate corruption. The problem: if it *is* corruption, it is hard to catch—or no politician would every do it. No one can blame politicians for receiving money towards their own political fortunes. But when people from these industries are placed in multiple positions of power, we should pause, notice.

A Vote for Trump is a Vote for a 2022 Mid-term Republican Disaster

In America, the power of government is supposed to be divided, according to the Constitution. There are checks and balances, to stop a President from becoming a king. Many are too young to remember "one party rule." It was extremely difficult for Republicans to regain control of the House of Representatives for 40 long years. Democrats outnumbered Republicans so much in the House, it took that many years to get it back. The personality, and actions of President Trump make such a sweep extremely likely in 2022.

President Trump complains all the time about Nancy Pelosi. Well, she became House leader in the 2018 midterms, because Republicans lost so many seats under Donald Trump. You are kidding yourself, if think President Trump's uncivilized mannerisms towards his enemies had nothing to do with this. Many Republicans accept this garbage, because he is winning their issues. But these victories will be short lived, according to the history of mid-term elections. Imagine the 2022 midterms if President Trump does something against the will of *90 percent* of the American people—like shut down medical cannabis.

---

281 W*ho Is Lobbying Mike Pence And Why? Health Insurers and Big Oil Seek To Influence Vice President.* By Alex Kotch. INTERNATIONAL BUSINESS TIMES. August 17, 2017

According to the memo he approved, this could happen.

In recent times, the party who controls the White House always loses Congressional seats in the midterms, with one exception. The severity of this loss depends on issues at the time. Last time, only the President's actions, and personality were a factor.

Next time, his personality will be an issue once again. Only without any fear of losing votes, he will not be restrained. And, he is restraining himself now, for that very purpose. What has damaged him, is what has slipped out of his mouth. "Out of the abundance of the heart, the mouth speaks[282]."

Republicans might have to have even more to deal with next time. If Trump shuts down the medical cannabis industry, the media will *have a field day.* If any epileptic dies—or anyone else with a serious medical condition—President Trump will be blamed. The families of real people will be interviewed. Everyone who became re-addicted to opiates—after cannabis is taken away—will have a story to tell. People will be in the streets protesting, because their votes became worthless because of Donald Trump.

Officials from local governments will be interviewed, talking about the loss of revenue from the industry shutdown, and all of the programs defunded. If President Trump is bull-headed enough to move against the will of the voters, he sets up this future political disaster. The *reason* will not matter; whether he wrongly believes cannabis causes a "permanent drop in IQ.,"Psychosis," "violence"—or because he is looking towards pharmaceutical remuneration after he leaves office. People will not rally around his cause as he believes—or thank him years later, after he "sets things straight." Instead, people will be mad their votes did not matter.

Both political parties play each other. Whether you are talking about the Republicans, or Democrats, *both* parties make it sound like it will be the "end of the world" if the other side wins. The reality? It takes government *a long time* for anything to get done. The government has not moved on cannabis reforms in 40 years, since the Shaffer commission recommended decriminalization. 8 years under Obama did *not* turn us into a socialist country as his detractors claimed.

Instead of reviewing the data of the Shaffer Commission, and following their recommendations to decriminalize cannabis, Richard Nixon bull-headily did what he thought was best, and ordered cannabis to be placed on Schedule 1. For years, people have suffered medically, financially, and legally because one man thought he knew best.

We are told the President views this issue like a father, to his children. The people are supposed to be represented in government, not led like sheep or small children. As Richard Nixon, President Trump is one man with a strong will that could hurt many people by ignoring the will of the voters, for what he thinks is best.

---

282 Proverbs 13:3; Luke 6:45

Addendum

A political "nuclear weapon" is not being used this election season, *and it should be.* This "weapon" is the issue of cannabis legalization:

"Undoubtedly vocalizing his support for legalization would draw voters in. "In 2018, top Democrats credited a legalization ballot initiative in Michigan with boosting turnout and producing the biggest blue wave in the country—winning races for governor, Senate, attorney general, and secretary of state, along with flipping two congressional seats and multiple state-legislature seats". Democrats are urging Biden to change his stance. "If Joe Biden's account tweeted out 'Legal. Weed.,' it would get a million likes in the first two hours. I guarantee it." - John Fetterman, the lieutenant governor of Pennsylvania." Cannabis could be an effective tool to win over voters from both sides of the aisle, so why is Joe Biden hesitant to join the rest of his party and most other Americans?" (The Marijuana Superweapon Biden Refuses to Use. By Edward-Isaac Dovere. THE ATLANTIC. July 6, 2020[283])

If you know a medical cannabis patient, who is also a Trump supporter, send them a copy of this book.

The E-book will get there quicker, and has links to follow, for further research. However, a hard copy is more likely to be read, especially if the person does not usually read. Also, an audio book will be available.

TrumpsHiddenAgenda.com

CBDSciencePortal.com

283 https://www.theatlantic.com/politics/archive/2020/07/biden-marijuana-pot-legalize/613777/

Other books by Russell Redden

Cannabis History, Law, and Health

THE REAL REASON CANNABIS HAS NOT BEEN RESCHEDULED: A CURE FOR CANCER DELAYED? 2017

THE MDK GENE AND CANNABIS AS A POTENTIAL CANCER CURE 2019

CBD AND THE CYTOKINE STORM: A POTENTIAL TREATMENT FOR COVID-19 OVERLOOKED? 2020

Theology Historic, Doctrine, Prophecy

Studies in Prophecy

Volume 1: **BEYOND COINCIDENCE: THE TESTIMONY OF PROPHECY** 2005

Volume 2: **RISE OF THE ASSYRIAN: THE ANTICHRIST, THE BEAST, AND THE REVIVED BABYLONIAN EMPIRE**
Second Edition 2008, Third Edition 2012
1st Edition: The Antichrist: Prince of Iraq 2006

Volume 3: **THE SEVENTH SHMITA: COUNTDOWN TO THE SECOND COMING** 2014

Studies in Theology

THE TIMELESS AGE OF GOD 2007

GENESIS AND JUBILEES: PARALLEL EDITION 2013

www.ingramcontent.com/pod-product-compliance
Lightning Source LLC
Chambersburg PA
CBHW061339250726
48657CB00004B/1240